[Cu]re: Your Fatigue

How balancing 3 minerals and 1 protein
Is the solution that you're looking for

[Cu]re: Your Fatigue

How balancing 3 minerals and 1 protein
Is the solution that you're looking for

Morley M. Robbins

gatekeeper press™

Columbus, Ohio

Disclaimer

The purpose of the book is to educate and to enlighten. It is not intended to serve as a replacement for professional medical advice. Any use of the information in this book is at the reader's discretion. This book is sold with the expressed understanding that neither the publisher nor the author has any liability or responsibility for any injury caused, or alleged to be caused. directly or indirectly, by the information contained in this book. While every effort has been made to ensure its accuracy, the book's contents should not be construed as medical advice. To obtain medical advice on your individual health needs, please consult a qualified health care practitioner.

Cu-RE Fatigue: The Root Cause and How To Fix It On Your Own

Published by Gatekeeper Press
2167 Stringtown Rd, Suite 109
Columbus, OH 43123-2989
www.GatekeeperPress.com

Library of Congress Control Number: 2021939216

ISBN (paperback): 9781662910289
eISBN: 9781662910296

This book is dedicated to:

Elizabeth Reed, DC

From the moment that I first met Dr. Liz, and she first spoke about the "*innate healer*," I was captivated to find out exactly who or what this internal healer really was... She knew it intuitively and intimately as a gifted natural healer, but she inspired me to learn about it physiologically, metabolically, and minerally. The world will never know her patience to endure my countless observations, over the course of a decade, about what each day's research findings were, nor her boundless ability to respond with: "*So what you're trying to say is...*" My hours and hours of relentless research routinely got reduced to a poignant, albeit powerful phrase, but she has consistently supported my quest, and has stimulated my desire to dig ever deeper... No one has ever loved me, nor has understood me, the way she does... I am forever grateful. She is the intentional, inspirational spark of my life.

Table of Contents

PART II: Action Steps To Create Greater Energy and Better Health

Acknowledgements

It is an absolute fact that this book would still be in my head were it not for the gift-of-gab talents of Larry Trivieri. He is known professionally as a ghostwriter, but I regard him as a friend and he volunteered to serve as my "guestwriter." I am deeply indebted to his unique ability to not just understand what I was seeking to say, but he learned to adopt my voice in crafting these many pages– a special talent that deserves greater recognition.

That said, I would be remiss in not also acknowledging the thousands of articles written by hundreds and hundreds of researchers that I have been graced to learn from. I can never identify all of them, but I will certainly highlight those that have had the deepest impact on my thinking and my understanding of how the human body really works, how it responds to stress and ultimately how this "stress response" affects our ability to make energy: Mildred S. Seelig, MD, MPH; Burton M. and Bella T. Altura, PhDs; Jean Durlach, MD; Frederick A. Kummerow, PhD; Leslie M. Klevay, MD, ScD; Jamie F. Collins, PhD; Marianne Wessling-Resnick, PhD; Mitchell D. Knutson, PhD; Susan S. Percival, PhD; Edward D. Harris, PhD; Guenther Weiss, MD; Joseph R. Prohaska, PhD; Robert R. Crichton, PhD; Paul A.

Cobine, PhD; Edward Weinberger, PhD; Jim Moon, PhD; Zena Leah Harris, MD; Weston A. Price, DDS; Gerald W. Deas, MD; Douglas B. Kell, PhD; Garth JS Cooper, DPh, DSc; Maxwell M. Wintrobe, MD, PhD; George E. Cartwright, MD; Svetlana Lutsenko, PhD, to name but a few... I am indeed humbled by the discipline and devotion with which these clinicians and researchers discovered and carried forth their message.

As we'll learn in the coming pages, it is not that their research hasn't been published. It simply is NOT being taught. Therein lies the origin of the "incomplete information" that shapes the thinking of practitioners responsible for healing on planet Earth.

In addition to these dedicated scientists who have guided and inspired me for a decade, I would remiss to not acknowledge and thank the thousands of members of the Magnesium Advocacy Facebook Group, the thousands of clients that I have had the privilege to work with, as well as the hundreds of individuals who have elected to be members of the RCP Community and/or complete the formal training of the RCP Institute to become RCP Consultants. This is an amazing body of talent that I am deeply inspired by and indebted to.

And finally, there are three very special people that deserve special recognition: Patrick Sullivan, Jr. (and the entire Sullivan family, for that matter...), Marilyn J. Hampstead, and most importantly, Kristan Kershaw. The RCP message, movement & MAG-nificance has been built on their passion to see these concepts reach a broader audience along with greater and greater levels of clarity and sophistication. Words fail me to express my heartfelt gratitude for all that they have done and continue to do, esp. the RCP Operations Executive, Kristan, for the countless hours of devotion and dedication to this program. "Thank you," works, but is hardly sufficient...

How to Use This Book...

This book is presented in two parts. First, the research basis for understanding how energy is made inside our bodies and how it is lost in our response to stress. The second is more of a practicum for how to apply the principles and process steps that have come to be known as the Root Cause Protocol.

As you might imagine, creating this book has been a labor of love, but it has also been a source of tremendous relief and recovery for those that have had a chance to partake of its unique nutritional focus. Please read this book as though your mind were a parachute – *most useful when open!* Much of what you "know" about your health condition, especially your fatigue, is flawed by "missing information." For those with a healthy skepticism that Copper is even a factor, or that copper and iron have a profound relationship with each other, I would encourage you to read:

- one ***very short*** article (Collins and Klevay, 2011) **https://academic.oup.com/advances/article/2/6/520/4664536?login=true**
- and one ***very long*** article (Doguer, Ha & Collins, 2018) **https://pubmed.ncbi.nlm.nih.gov/30215866/**

These will be available on the dedicated website: **https:// cureyourfatiguebook.com/resources**

The breadth, depth and range of footnotes of this latter article are a *tour-de-force* that should offer even the greatest skeptic sufficient proof that we have been Misled and Misfed about the ancient and dynamic relationship between these two very primal and powerful redox metals.

Absent this key information regarding these key metals, we lack the truth of human physiology. Please use this book as a resource to challenge your belief system, but also as a stimulus to learn to ask better questions, and most importantly, to learn to demand better answers.

Ideally, I would like to see this book not only become a resource for both overcoming your fatigue, but also your dependence on others to "heal" you. Our ultimate goal, in my humble opinion, is to learn to take control of the process to attain our health freedom, and thereby ensure that we gain our medical independence.

Introduction

by Ben Edwards, MD

The book you are about to read is going to challenge everything you may know or think you know about diet, nutrition, health, and disease. I can say that because the information it contains certainly challenged me when I first encountered it. It ran contrary to everything I previously understood about the real cause of fatigue— the number one health complaint patients make to their doctors— and, more importantly, the real cause of the vast majority of diseases that afflict so many people today. Rather than rejecting this new information, I decided to delve into it further. I'm very glad I did, because applying what you are about to learn in this book has enabled me to understand the "root cause" of my patients' health challenges and provided me with the tools I need to most properly address them, leading my patients back to good health.

Let me explain.

I think deep down most physicians know and accept the fact that, when it comes to health and disease, diet and lifestyle are two of the most significant determining factors. That's even what the medical research says these days. Cancer, diet, and lifestyle. Heart disease, diet, and lifestyle. The research also points to inflammation as being these conditions' common denominator. That's really starting to come out of the literature now. If you're talking autism, Alzheimer's, or depression, that's brain inflammation. Coronary artery disease is a disease of inflammation. Cancer is a disease of inflammation. And, of course, all the autoimmune diseases are obviously diseases of inflammation, as well.

There's an ongoing inflammatory process that's happening more and more among our population and becoming chronic. And it's occurring more frequently even among younger and younger age groups. What most physicians, including myself, have been trained to do is prescribe drugs to try to tamp down that inflammatory cascade. But what we haven't trained enough in is how to look deeper to find a root cause for this inflammatory cascade and the subsequent lack of energy and eventual disease that it leads to. Nutrition is a big part of this. And a big part of what is missing in medical schools.

When I think back to my education at the University of Texas Health Science Center at Houston, I realize I only received about one to two hours of nutrition training during my entire four years of medical school. I remember an elective nutrition course I attended. It was not part of the main curriculum. It was an elective presented at lunchtime. About twenty of my fellow students and I showed up because they had free pizza. There was a cardiologist putting slides up on the board about the reversal of coronary artery disease, also known as ischemia. He had these profusion scans, pre and post. And his treatment wasn't statins and beta blockers. It was nutrition. That fascinated me. I asked him, "Why are we hearing this at a lunchtime elective lecture when hardly anybody is here? Why isn't what you presented part of the main curriculum?"

I will never forget his reply:

"Well, there's a lot of money to be had in bypass surgeries and stents, and there's not a lot of money to be had in teaching someone how to eat."

Now fast forward. I had a patient who came to me suffering from a number of chronic diseases. I was able to help her manage some of her symptoms, but although my treatment plan for her provided relief, her symptoms persisted.

A few months later, she followed up with me and told she had found something online that was helping her. Now, patients come in all the time and tell their doctors they read something online that they hope might help them. As physicians, knowing the glut of worthless and even potentially harmful information that is online, we can tell very quickly if what the patients find is something to pay attention to or not. Almost always, it isn't, and we have to tell our patients that they can't and shouldn't believe everything they see on the internet. In short, we blow it off.

But this time was different. This woman had started to follow the dietary and nutritional protocol that she had found online—*the same ones that you are about to discover in this book*—and even though it had only been a few months since my last appointment with her, I could tell that she was a new woman. Her depression, her chronic fatigue syndrome, and all of the other kinds of vague symptoms that we don't like to deal with as doctors because we don't have a good answer for them, were all significantly improved. And her energy levels had also soared. She was dramatically different from when I'd last seen her. She was well.

This greatly intrigued me because I went to medical school to help people, and I wasn't able to help her. Yet, there she was sitting in front of me saying she followed this protocol she found on the internet and because of it she was better.

Now some doctors might have shrugged off such a positive turnaround in their patients. Unfortunately, it's not uncommon for doctors to not look further into what causes such a result. At best, they might say, "*Well, whatever it is you are doing seems to be working, so keep doing it,*" but that's where their curiosity ends.

I'm not like that. I'm all ears when it comes to anything that can be shown to have helped fatigued and ill patients because I realized years ago that we physicians have reached a plateau in our ability to manage chronic disease and get results using the conventional tools of our trade. There's got to be something more to health care than symptom-management using pharmaceutical drugs. I know that diet has an impact. I know lifestyle and stress management do too. But until this woman's turnaround, I did not know much of anything about what had helped her get better so quickly. Although reversing major diseases was not foreign to me, it was a real challenge to know how to handle the tougher cases or non-responders. Medical school taught me how to reduce their symptoms and related ailments, but not how to reverse them. Integrative and functional medicine also helped to some extent because it helped reduce some inflammation through diet and lifestyle changes. But, when she showed me the protocol she was following, I did go online to read about it and began to seriously consider it. And that's when I learned about Morley Robbins and how the Root Cause Protocol he pioneered and continues to fine tune was helping not only my patient, but so many other people who previously for years had also been coping with chronic fatigue and many other chronic health conditions.

Since my initial exposure to his work, Morley and I have become both friends and colleagues, and I have incorporated the Root Cause Protocol into my medical practice because I know it works. I have also joined with Morley to oversee the RCP Institute, which offers a 14-week training course for physicians and other health practitioners, as well as lay people, interested in entering the health field as health coaches and RCP consultants. I only wish I'd had this training available to me when I was in medical school!

What I find most interesting about Morley, who is not a doctor, is that, because of his commitment to sleuthing out the underlying mechanisms that have led to the massive explosion of chronic disease in the United States and around the world, he has spent the past ten years digging into the peer-reviewed medical journals, examining the research and "connecting the dots" in a manner that has never been done before. To that end, Morley spends a minimum of two to three hours every morning, seven days a week, combing through the research. The knowledge and understanding he has gained by doing so is what impressed me the most when I first met him. Not only was he able to clearly communicate what he believes is the root cause of fatigue, chronic inflammation, and disease, he backed it up with the thousands of research studies and articles he's pored through and studied.

Unfortunately, there exists a bias among the medical community, researchers, and our nation's health organizations at the federal, state, and local levels. That bias favors the type and amount of education we doctors receive in medical school. That, in turn, keeps the focus narrowed on conventional, drug-based treatments and little else. But there is a broader way to look at the human body, and to look at disease management and even reversal of disease, when we start delving deeper into the root cause.

Type 2 diabetes is a great example. We're chasing blood sugars all day long, using drugs like metformin and insulin shots and so forth. But the actual cause is insulin resistance. We know this, but we just continue treating elevated blood sugar. That's very much like treating a fever with Tylenol when you have a gangrenous wound on the leg. Tylenol may reduce a 100-degree fever down to 98.6, but we all understand that it is not the right course of action for treating gangrene. The root cause of the fever is the infection. We need to deal with that. The root cause of the high blood sugar is insulin resistance. We need to deal with that, as well. Yet, it turns out there is just not a medication that really deals with insulin resistance. The medications only deal with blood sugar.

So, although the information you are about to read is different from what you may already know, and certainly different from what doctors and other health practitioners are taught in medical school, I invite you to read it with an open mind. I think we can all agree that what we're doing now is not working. We're a sick country. The disease burdens on our nation are skyrocketing. As Morley likes to say, we've all been *"misled and misfed."* What is needed to reverse this trend is a deeper, more comprehensive level of understanding of chronic disease and more fundamentally, the energy loss in the body that causes it. I believe that Morley has found it.

But don't take my word for it. This book is designed primarily to provide you with the information you need to begin applying the Root Cause Protocol immediately. In Part One, you will learn what Morley has discovered and how health, fatigue, and disease are all dependent primarily on the interrelated dynamic, or "dance", of three minerals—magnesium, copper, and iron—and their levels and bioavailability in your body. In Part Two, you will learn the practical applications of Morley's discoveries and how to put them to use. Once you start to do so, you will be on the way to proving for yourself how well the Root Cause Protocol really works. Your fatigue will begin to fade away and be replaced by levels of energy you might never have thought possible for yourself. I encourage you to begin that journey right now.

A Word to Skeptics

For you physicians and other readers with a scientific bent, I realize the temptation you may have to ignore the rest of this book because of what I wrote above. You may be thinking, *The key to the Root Cause Protocol is basically three minerals? Nonsense! How can it be that simple?* I understand such skepticism because I once shared it. In fact, I applaud skepticism as an appropriate response when it comes to new health claims. But there is a big difference between being a skeptic and being a cynic unwilling to consider challenges to one's cherished beliefs. Cynics, I find, tend to simply reject new ideas and possibilities out of hand. Skeptics, by contrast, welcome the chance to investigate new ideas and possibilities, putting them to the test. And if they find they work and are real, they are also willing to change their minds—for their benefit and for the benefit of their fellow human beings.

That's why I invite those who want to pursue the science that backs Morley's findings in more detail to seek out and read the many scientific studies that Morley has included in this book. You will discover medical research and studies from around the world, conducted as far back as 1910 right up to the present, all synthesized together by Morley. As I've said, he's spent years connecting the dots, and once you read through these studies, I'm confident you won't be able to deny what the research is pointing to. I think you'll find it both very educational and eye-opening.

And now, as Morley is also fond of saying,

A vôtre santé! (To your health!)

Ben Edwards, MD is an integrative physician, member of the Academy of Comprehensive Integrative Medicine (ACIM), and the founder and medical director of Veritas Medical in Lubbock, Texas, as well as serving on the medical advisory board of the RCP Institute.

Foreward

by Brice T. Smith, MD

I must confess to a long-standing interest in nutrition ("bio-hacking" would actually be the better term). Over many years, after much trial and error, I eventually discovered a few supplements that proved essential in my high-stress profession. But before learning of Morley Robbins's work, I had abandoned hope of finding a unifying theory of nutrition. Even so, I kept an eye out for one that not only identified key nutritional factors, but also one that placed dietary supplements in a reasonable hierarchy. Since a new paradigm failed to appear, I just kept trying new things without much direction, driven as much by hype as by fact.

Long before I met him, my first impression about Morley was, "How about that? Morley tells you what to stop before doing anything else!" If you can't do something good, at least stop doing something bad. In the last year, Morley and I have been fortunate to have had many long discussions. I believe he has become proficient in his subject in a way that few others could, physician or not.

The topics you will read about in this book, based on Morley's discoveries, are so huge that they might overwhelm you, even as they tend to overwhelm me, were they not streamlined for consumption. Whereas many nutritional claims are backed up by reference to one lone medical paper or study, Morley can cite multiple studies for every point he makes, and at least one of these will be a landmark, game-changing study. He has ventured down numerous rabbit holes where few are likely to follow. One might say he is obsessed, but it is because of his persistent inquiries that he now commands a vast quantity of biochemical and physiological data. He is able to discuss in detail how all this biochemistry is connected, how it becomes afflicted, how equilibrium might best be restored, which things are critical, and which are not that important, and ultimately, what is flat out wrong! This is the hierarchy of nutritional understanding that I have been looking for since the mid-1980s!

The most intelligent person I ever met was a physics major back in college. Problem solving was easy for him. "I just convert everything into the energy frame of reference, and the answer falls out," he told me. Sounds easy, right?

Morley has taken his time and knowledge and condensed it into this same energy frame of reference. His hope (and mine as well) is that it will help to fix the fatigue and outright exhaustion that seems to plague most members of our society.

The fix does not require that you to do a decade of your own research, nor decades of trial and error, merely that you implement some good advice. The answer has fallen out, and is now in your hands. Ignore it at your peril.

Brice T. Smith, MD is a radiologist in Chapel Hill, North Carolina. He received his medical degree from Uniformed Services University of the Health Sciences and has been in practice for more than 35 years.

Preface

by Karen Lemacks Gadol, PA-C, RCPC

I have been a student of Morley Robbins since 2017, and a follower of his work for years before that. We met for the first time in an elevator in Chicago at a Health Freedom Expo in 2013. I had traveled there with friends specifically to hear him speak. When I got on the elevator and saw him there, I introduced myself as a "fan". We rode down the elevator together – just the two of us – and had a brief conversation as we traveled down to the conference floor. I'm very pleased to say the he (and his wife Dr. Liz) are now my friends and he is a mentor whom I trust and respect.

I've been a traditionally-trained licensed practitioner (PA-C) for over 20 years. I "stepped out of the box" in 2009 when I started to get sick (I now understand it was due to much stress and the mineral dysregulation it causes) and I've never looked back. The more I learn, the more I learn I don't know. I'm so happy to also share that today I am well and able to share the TRUTHS that you are about to read about with others.

I will say that although the protocol's steps are simple, the scientific basis for each of them is straightforward, but not necessarily easy. The human body is wonderfully made with many levels of activity. What happens at the cellular level and our mineral intake determines our health status, vitality, and longevity as you are about to discover. But, don't let the profound intricacies of human biology overwhelm you. I've been studying these topics for over four years and on many occasions, I still have to reread details and sentences to truly grasp the concepts discussed.

So, please be encouraged. If you are committed to improving your well-being, but aren't necessarily interested in diving into the details of the supporting scientific evidence, that's perfectly fine. In any case, I urge you to begin following the RCP. Based upon my years of experience with the program, I assure you that your health can only improve from its guidance!

Morley is extremely intelligent and deeply committed to helping others. I learn from him every day, and I'm honored to call him a friend.I believe you will have the same experience by reading the book you hold in your hands. Enjoy it and be well!

Karen Lemacks Gadol, PA-C, is physician's assistant in Mt. Pleasant, SC. She is a certified professional cancer coach, thermographer and RCP consultant. She is also the creator of iDetox, http://theirontruth.com

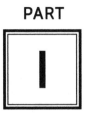

Why You're So Tired

Misled and Misfed

"Whenever you find yourself on the side of the majority, it is time to pause and reflect."
– Samuel Clemens (Mark Twain)

"Pasteur's mechanistic understanding of disease took away the individual's power to prevent it, and placed the mandate to cure squarely in the hands of the medical professionals."
– Ron Schmid, ND (1946 – 2017)

You most likely picked up this book because you are suffering from persistent fatigue and you're tired of it. You want a solution, something that works that will enable you to regain your energy and improve your overall health.

If this describes you, you are not alone. As Dr. Edwards stated in this book's Introduction, fatigue is the most common health complaint patients report to their physicians. But as Dr. Edwards also indicated, few physicians today know what to do to help their patients banish fatigue. To know how to truly do this is simply not in their wheelhouse. Shocking and sad, isn't it?

In the pages that follow, I am going to tell you why that is. More importantly, I am going to tell you how energy in your body is produced and what you can and must do to ensure that it is produced properly and abundantly so that before long the fatigue that is plaguing you is banished once and for all. Best of all, I am going to show you how to make this happen simply and easily, all on your own. I wrote this book so that you and your loved ones can join the many thousands of other people whose health and energy levels have turned around by putting to use the same information you are about to learn, which I call the Root Cause Protocol because it addresses the real root, or underlying, cause that is keeping you tired and lacking vibrant health.

What The Root Cause Protocol Can Do For You

What follow are but a few examples of what is possible for you. They are testimonials I've received from people just like you who turned their lives around by following the same recommendations you will find in this book. (For the sake of their privacy, only their first names are used.)

For 21 years, Therese suffered from Lyme disease along with rickettsias, a type of intracellular, parasitic bacteria. During all of that time, her condition continued to worsen.

Two years before discovering the Root Cause Protocol, she began following the Body Ecology Diet while attempting to work "nearly full-time." Rather than experiencing an improvement in her symptoms, Therese reports, "I became super unwell. The cultured vegetables [pickled or fermented vegetables that are a centerpiece of the Body Ecology Diet] were making me very ill, and in the end they caused a thyroid problem for me, along with other spiraling problems." Because of the diet, Therese also suspected she was lacking enough omega-3 essential fatty acids, along with various minerals.

Fortunately, a friend she knew told Therese about the Root Cause Protocol. Therese discussed it with her doctor, who told her she thought there would be no harm in Therese trying it. After Therese began the Root Cause Protocol, she wrote, "I started Phase 2 of the Root Cause Protocol about a week ago and just this past week I've really noticed I'm feeling better in energy levels and stamina. This is all amazing as I've only been doing RCP for two months!

It's marvelous and I know it's helping me."

Like Therese, Liv had also suffered poor health and persistent fatigue for many years.

This is the testimonial she shared with me one year after she adopted the Root Cause Protocol: "Tomorrow marks an exciting day for me because it will have been a year since I stopped metabolic Thyroid Rx medication after using it for 17 years. This last year hasn't been a roller coaster because it has only gone all the way up. I have simply balanced the minerals in the body, and ensured that magnesium, iron, copper, zinc and calcium have become more balanced. I have increased my ceruloplasmin production so that iron and copper are moving in my body, and are not stored in my organs and tissues. In November of last year, I had a ferritin level of 126. Today, my ferritin level is at 18. They haven't been that low in decades.

"I do things I haven't done in years, and have energy left when the working day is over to do things other than just work. These last months have been busy, both with work and in private, and my spare time goes to things it didn't before, like going skiing and taking trips to the mountains. I'm doing things I once thought I would never be able to do again. My God, how wonderful it is to feel like you're alive! I will forever be grateful for you, Morley Robbins and for everything you have taught me."

You will soon learn what ceruloplasmin is and why balancing the minerals Liv mentions are so important. First, here are a few more testimonials that illustrate what the Root Cause Protocol can possibly do for you.

Dale is a 54-year-old man who suffered from "unshakable weariness, tiredness, and lack of energy" for years. After adopting the Root Cause Protocol, he states, "Two years on, I feel much improved. My feeling of well-being is so much better. I am learning a huge amount from Morley and the research that he unveils. Clearly, achieving the correct balance of minerals and nutrients no doubt varies from one person to another, but I have found the Root Cause Protocol easy to follow and the rewards have come relatively swiftly for me. Morley's tireless research is very much appreciated."

Jane began implementing the Root Cause Protocol out of frustration after numerous medical tests failed to help her. As she put it, "I've had X-rays, ultrasounds, and enough blood tests to fill an entire person trying to get to the bottom of what the hell was wrong with me. But when I went to the doctor today, I couldn't contain my excitement.

"After discovering the Root Cause Protocol, I've been focusing on getting my magnesium intake up, and purging unbound iron. As a result, the swelling in my feet is gone, my leg and calf cramps are gone, my restless leg syndrome is gone, and my insomnia and heart palpitations are gone. My anxiety is practically gone, as well. I have so much more energy. I feel ten years younger. I'm not waking up fatigued. I feel incredible, I'm riding my horse again and I'm going to work happy! My doctor typed furiously as I spoke, and then sat there stunned, with a big grin on her face, and told me how pleased she was for me."

Linette is another person who suffered from Lyme disease, persistent fatigue her doctors ascribed to anemia, and other health issues. After following the Root Cause Protocol for seven months, she wrote, "When I started to dig deeper in researching natural protocols for Lyme healing, I came across the Root Cause Protocol via the Magnesium Advocacy Group on Facebook. It has been the best thing ever! Previous to finding this, I had only portions of truth that would help. I've tried every detox, every cleanse, and been to so many doctors and naturopaths, to little avail. I prayed that God would send me to the right path. My whole life I have been told I was anemic. But now I know the truth! Thank God for Morley and his leadership.

"You cannot go wrong with the Root Cause Protocol. Your thyroid, hormones, pain, inflammation, weakness, restless legs, sleeplessness, nervousness, and more can all be helped. I am living proof. I'm telling all of my friends and acquaintances with Lyme, fibromyalgia, chronic fatigue, thyroid issues, and adrenal issues to get on the Root Cause Protocol. Now they are feeling better also.

"My life was not even worth living at one point. I now am exercising, getting my strength back, and can tolerate stress! I cannot express how happy and thankful I am."

Finally, here is a message I received from Staci. "Being on the Root Cause Protocol for just over three months has completely changed my life. I feel so good, sleep so well, have energy that I've not known since high school, and am more focused, yet relaxed, than ever in my life. I sometimes feel bionic. I am 46 years old. I feel 25. It is blowing my mind."

Naturally, I am very happy with the results the people above and thousands of others have achieved by using the Root Cause Protocol. At the same time, though, I lament the fact that countless millions of other people continue to struggle with fatigue and a wide range of chronic degenerative health conditions. Why is this so? Why aren't their doctors truly able to help them instead of just prescribing them with drugs that, at best, do little more than manage, not reverse, their symptoms, and at worse (and very likely) cause serious side effects that make their patients even sicker? Why is it that the vast majority of doctors do not know what I know, when I'm not a doctor and they've had, at minimum, eight years of medical education? Why is it that all disease begins with a loss of energy? What is the truth about the answers to such questions? Allow me to tell you.

My Story

Given that I am **not** a doctor, you may be wondering how and why
I came to research minerals and ultimately discover each of the life
changing elements of the Root Cause Protocol.

Well, first of all, I do have a mainstream medical industry
background, having been a hospital executive and consultant for
32 years. My journey beyond that paradigm began several years ago
and it all started with my shoulder. More specifically, it began when
I developed a condition called "frozen shoulder," following 20 years
of dragging a suitcase behind my back.

When I went to see my doctor about my painful right arm, he
quickly recommended surgery as my only hope if I wanted to be able
to lift my right hand above my waist ever again. Surgery didn't appeal
to me, so I put it off. Then, friends of mine who owned a health food
store encouraged me to try chiropractic care. My initial response
to them, which illustrates how little I actually knew about health
and healing back then, was, *"Thanks guys, but I don't do witchcraft."*
Instead, I stubbornly suffered with my condition for several more
months.

Finally, my friends had enough of my stubbornness and insisted
I see a chiropractor.

Because the pain I was in continued to wear on me, I finally
agreed. After only a couple weeks of light touch chiropractic care in
the form of a technique known as Network Spinal Analysis, I was
stunned to find my shoulder had regained its full range of motion
once again, and my pain was all but gone.

That experience was so life-changing for me, that I began
questioning everything I knew—or thought I knew—about healing.
Soon thereafter, I left the world of hospital administration and dove
deep down the rabbit hole, determined to discover what true healing,
not symptom care, actually involved. I was guided by two burning

questions: ***Why are so many people everywhere so sick today?*** And, the corollary question, which came later: ***Why are so many people so fatigued and told they have anemia when we exist on a planet that is ~35 percent iron?***

I started to find the answers to those questions in July 2009, when I read Carolyn Dean's wonderful book *The Magnesium Miracle*. I realized that the information she shared within it was a key piece of the whole health puzzle that virtually no physicians or other health care practitioners seemed to be aware of, including doctors within the worlds of alternative, integrative, and functional medicine. I was captivated by this mineral, and went on to read even more. Much more.

Thirty-five books and over 6,000 articles about mineral deficiencies and mineral dysregulation later, I knew for certain that magnesium plays a vital role in all of the body's metabolic systems, and that magnesium deficiency, which virtually all people today suffer from, is therefore a major contributing factor to nearly all major health issues. In fact, based on all of the scientific studies I pored through, I realized that magnesium deficiency, or insufficiency, is at the center of all these common modern diseases due to its central role in activating 3,751 proteins (Piovesan et al, 2012), and thus thousands of enzyme systems (far more than the common online and published figure of 300 enzyme pathways, as Burt Vallee, MD, of Harvard Medical School pointed out in a 1955 interview).

So, for a time, I made it my life's work to push back the tides of nutritional insanity by informing as many people as I could about magnesium deficiency in their day-to-day lives, and, more importantly, how they could rectify that problem and help end the epidemic of magnesium deficiency that is plaguing the health and well-being of Western civilization. To that end, in 2012, I founded the Magnesium Advocacy Facebook group, which currently has almost 200,000 members, and continues to grow by the hundreds weekly.

I have also completed training for becoming a Wellness Coach, a Nutritional Counselor, and a Functional Diagnostic Nutritionist, with an expertise in Hair Tissue Mineral Analysis (HTMA), a very important, yet little used, health assessment test that we will learn more about in Part Two of this book.

However, despite all that I knew about the importance of magnesium, my desire to keep learning all I could in order to help people regain their energy and health compelled me to keep "digging deeper" into the scientific literature. As I did so, I discovered that magnesium, while still being a primary cornerstone in the foundation of true health, was not the entire solution. And that's when the corollary question I mentioned earlier really began to take hold of me. I knew that magnesium was extremely important—absolutely essential, in fact—for combating fatigue and producing more energy, but as I continued to consult with those seeking my help, I could not escape the fact that, even after they followed my advice and improved their bodies' magnesium stores, not everyone was able to banish fatigue. I was determined to find out why that was.

So, deeper and deeper, I kept digging. And what I discovered after more years of doing so is that the answers I was looking for all have to do with a protein/enzyme most people have never heard of, called **ceruloplasmin**. The more I study this protein, the more fascinated I am by its role, functions, and diverse activity in our metabolism. What I've learned is that the lack of ceruloplasmin prevents our bodies from being able to metabolize iron (Holmberg and Laurell, 1948; Osaki et al, 1966; Roeser et al, 1970). And this iron-ic dynamic, in turn, creates oxidative stress, which is at the root of both persistent fatigue and chronic disease. This relentless process of oxidative stress is also the metabolic cause of the ubiquitous loss of magnesium.

That's not all I discovered. And when I say "discovered," I don't mean to say or imply that I am the first person to make this discovery. *Not at all!* The actual and original discoverers have been laying out these truths in the medical literature for nearly 100 years (McHargue et al, 1925; Hart et al, 1928), only to have their findings ignored. I will explain why shortly. In addition to magnesium and ceruloplasmin, there are two other key players inside your body that directly influence your health for better or worse: copper and iron. You are going to learn a lot more about all four of these elements in the rest of this book. For now, please remember this: Contrary to what almost all doctors believe and tell their patients, copper is not toxic and, if you are chronically-fatigued, you are not anemic but, for a fact, suffer from iron dysfunction, NOT iron deficiency. This misunderstanding of iron dynamics is a true global pandemic.

In actuality, you most likely have too much iron in your cells, tissues and organs, and not enough bioavailable copper available to do its job of regulating iron metabolism. The truth of the matter is that copper is missing in action and iron becomes stuck in the cells! Because copper is missing, that's why the iron gets stuck in your tissues and doesn't show up in your blood, and this iron in the tissue can be up to ten times the amount in our blood. (Killilea and Ames, 2004).

Please remember this, in particular: There's an enormous difference between the iron circulating in our blood versus the iron deposited into our organs and other tissues. Furthermore, we've got to stop believing that the iron level in our blood is perfectly representative of iron that's accumulated within our organs and other tissues. **It is not.** And when copper is missing in action and iron becomes trapped, utterly useless and toxic in our organs and other tissue cells, it becomes dysfunctional (Weiss and Goodnough, 2005; Wessling-Resnick, 2010; Gulec and Collins, 2014).

Research dating all the way back to 1928 proves that the **lack of bioavailable copper causes iron accumulation in the tissues**, especially in the liver (Hart et al, 1928; Elvehjem & Sherman, 1932). It is this lack of bioavailable copper in our daily diet that forces our body to accumulate iron where it doesn't belong (Gutteridge and Halliwell, 1984), thus causing the cascade of cellular and mitochondrial oxidative stress events that is keeping you fatigued and setting the stage for chronic conditions (Harman, 1956; 1972; 2006). That, in my humble opinion, is one of the most unique, most important, and most overlooked qualities of human metabolism.

The scientific, peer-reviewed literature from around the world—though not well known in conventional medical circles—is quite clear, consistent, and compelling. Persistent fatigue, as well as all disease, is caused by oxidative stress. And the root cause of oxidative stress is "cellular dysfunction" caused by an imbalance of three key minerals: copper, iron, and thus magnesium, compounded by a lack of ceruloplasmin, which prevents our ability to metabolize energy, recycle iron in the mitochondria, and, therefore, prevent harm caused by iron's inevitable interactions with oxygen in our tissues and blood. Copper harnesses oxygen, in much the same way that a chef harnesses the ingredients s/he uses when cooking and creating a delicious meal, as well as a dietary experience. Iron's function, by contrast, is to transport oxygen in much the same way that a waiter carries the meal to the diners in a restaurant. Eighty percent of the body's stores of iron are "carrying oxygen," but the real action occurs in the copper-directed "kitchens," called our mitochondria. And please keep in mind, despite our banter and relationship with the waiter, the REAL reason we go to restaurants is for the chef-inspired nutritional experience originating in that kitchen!

Seventy percent of the iron in the body exists as hemoglobin, and another ten percent of iron exists as myoglobin in the muscle. By restoring the proper balance of these three minerals and increasing the bioavailability of copper via the action of ceruloplasmin, you can feel much better by following the steps of the Root Cause Protocol. I wrote this book to teach you how to do so.

All of this is explained in more detail, beginning in Chapter 2. Now that you know my story, let's move on.

Misled and Misfed

I've spent over a decade of my life now unraveling the story of magnesium, copper, iron, and ceruloplasmin and how they are designed by nature to interact to maintain our health, as well as what happens when these interactions are interfered with, primarily as a result of following the accepted, yet highly flawed health recommendations we are all too familiar with.

At best, these recommendations are the result of ongoing human errors on the part of the medical profession, government health agencies, commercial farming and food manufacturing industries, dieticians and most nutritionists, and even proponents of nutritional supplements. At worst, they may be due to a more nefarious agenda, one designed to prevent us from achieving the optimal health and abundant energy we all deserve. Overall, I've come to recognize that it's the first factor—lack of curiosity and human error—that is mostly responsible for the health care crisis our nation and other nations face. And getting—and staying—angry about it serves little purpose, beyond triggering the body's stress response, which in turn can rapidly deplete its mineral stores, especially its magnesium status. Still, becoming aware of the ways in which we as a populace have been misled and misfed, whether intentionally or not, is vitally important if we are to find our way back to the truth.

Looking Into The Distant Past To Understand The Present: Everybody wants to know *"what's new?"* Truth be told, I've learned (from a day I spent with a brilliant marketing consultant) that it's far more important to understand *"what's enduring?"* I consider the biggest overlooked clue to understanding fatigue to be what happened when oxygen first began to accumulate in the

Earth's atmosphere long, long ago. According to astrophysicists, this occurred approximately 2.45 billion years ago and is referred to as the Great Oxygen Event (GOE), which is also referred to as the Oxygen Catastrophe or the Oxygen Holocaust because of how its occurrence caused 99 percent of the existing species on Earth to die out (Crichton & Pierre, 2001). Prior to this time, Earth's atmosphere was what is called a reducing atmosphere, an atmospheric condition is which oxidation (rusting) is prevented by natural mechanisms that removed oxygen, the primary one being iron oxides in both the land and the oceans. This removal process is known as "mass rusting." That's the first part of the clue.

Why? Because the oxidative stress in the body that saps energy and causes disease also causes our tissues and organs to "rust."

The vast majority of species alive on Earth before the GOE were anaerobic, meaning they did not require oxygen to survive. The oceans were much shallower than they are today. Then, species known as cyanobacteria, which contain copper that facilitates energy from oxygen photosynthesis, began releasing oxygen as a waste product into the atmosphere, eventually to such a degree that there was enough iron oxide to capture all of the oxygen that was being released into the atmosphere. A mere one percent accumulation of oxygen in the atmosphere is what caused the GOE. And since oxygen is toxic to anaerobic species, they were wiped out because they had no way to deal with the oxygen buildup. Prior to the GOE, the Earth's atmosphere contained only one-tenth of one percent (0.1 percent) oxygen, yet the increase to one percent is estimated to have wiped out 99 percent of all life on the planet (Crichton & Pierre, 2001; Kaplan & O'Halloran, 1996). Given this ancient devastation, it is far easier to understand that, next to fluoride, oxygen is regarded as the most reactive element on planet Earth. Yes, it is toxic to aerobic beings, as well. And that basic biological truth is not properly taught in doctor school.

So how was it that life on the planet was not eliminated altogether?

The answer and the second part of the clue is that copper literally saved the day and saved life as we know it. Once the GOE occurred, the planet, so long used to operating anaerobically, now had to find a way to deal with oxygen. After all, oxygen is the second most reactive element on the planet after fluorine. Copper, along with the enzymes that it expresses through, one class of which are known as multi-copper oxidases (and there are over a thousand different forms of them on the planet), solved this problem because of copper's unique ability to turn one molecule of oxygen into two molecules of water (O_2 into $2H_2O$) without producing any oxidative "exhaust" (Vaschenko et al, 2013). That is the gift of copper to our planet, and also to our physiology. We need bioavailable copper to prevent oxidative stress. which it does by transforming oxygen into water or into other usable metabolites in our bodies.

Today, the Earth's atmosphere is composed of nearly 21 percent oxygen. Were it not for copper, life on Earth would be impossible. In fact, all life on this planet must have copper to survive. (Published interview with Paul A. Cobine, PhD, 2017.) Similarly, without enough bioavailable copper in our body, oxygen by its reactive nature will inexorably begin to damage our tissue and our mitochondria, ultimately depleting our energy production and eventually destroying our health. Copper, when naturally working through its network of enzymes, is the only element in the body that works with oxygen cleanly to prevent oxygen from "rusting out" our cells, tissues, and organs. In addition, copper is the only element that regulates iron's status, thus preventing its reactions with oxygen that inevitably leads to this "rusting" process! When oxygen cannot be activated by copper in our mitochondria, to make water, to release energy molecules (Mg-ATP), it results in oxidative stress, aka free radicals, reactive oxygen species (ROS), and oxidants. This supports the "Free Radical Theory of Aging" first proposed by Denham Harman, PhD, MD

(1956; 1972; 2006) which is the most accepted model for aging, and is a major cornerstone of my counter-intuitive and counter-cultural thinking, which we will explore further in Chapter 5.

The third part of the clue is also well worth paying attention to. At almost the same time that the GOE occurred, cholesterol first made its appearance. That's right, cholesterol's appearance on the planet goes nearly all the way back to the beginning of oxygen's appearance (Galea & Brown, 2009; Brown & Galea, 2010). And, contrary to still popular, misguided (and, therefore, myth-leading) opinion, cholesterol is not a toxin, a disease product, nor the cause of disease. In fact, it takes 11 molecules of oxygen to make one molecule of cholesterol. So cholesterol is really an oxygen sink for an organism that doesn't have enough copper to activate the oxygen to make energy (Mg-ATP) in the mitochondria or to de-activate the oxidants (accidents with oxygen) to prevent oxidative stress. For billions of years, cholesterol has helped all such organisms to survive, including we human beings ever since we first appeared on the planet. Among its many functions, cholesterol acts as a governor to regulate how much oxygen passes through the cell membranes into the cells (Zuniga-Hertz et al, 2019; Klevay LM, 1973). The less bioavailable copper you have, the more your body will produce oxidative stress, which will then cause an increase in cholesterol levels for this very reason. And that rising oxidative stress will "rust" the cholesterol. It was never about the level of cholesterol. It was always about the amount of iron.

So what do these clues tell us? First of all, they tell us that, until the supply of oxygen began to increase, iron (in the form of iron oxides) and oxygen levels were kept at bay by mass rusting. Note that the iron oxides were inert, meaning they were bound to the land and oceans, where they captured and held onto oxygen. How does that relate to your health? Very simply: Inert, or bound iron, in your tissues and organs also captures oxygen, causing them to "rust" or oxidize. In order to be healthy and have all of the energy you need, instead of being bound in the tissues, iron in our body needs to be mobilized and circulating, so that it can carry oxygen to all of our organs, tissues, cells, and ultimately to the mitochondria to be turned into energy. That is what iron is designed to do – deliver more oxygen. But once it becomes immobilized and bound (stuck) in tissues, health problems begin as the levels of oxidative stress rise from failed energy production and failed oxidant elimination (Wessling-Resnick & Knutson, 2004; Collins, Prohaska & Knutson, 2010).

That's why copper is so important. Just as it rescued life on the planet billions of years ago, so too is it safeguarding our health so long as we do all that is necessary to enable it to do so (following the Root Cause Protocol is a key foundation).

The first principle to understand if you want to regain your energy and improve your health is that if we humans can't work with oxygen, we've got a major metabolic problem. Copper, acting on this first principle, acts with oxygen to do two things. First, it activates oxygen to create water that then releases energy, and then it deactivates oxidants (accidents with oxygen) to clear metabolic exhaust. That's the unique gift of copper. It has the ability to create energy inside our cells' "energy factories," which we call mitochondria, through the key enzyme called cytochrome c-oxidase (Complex IV of the electron transport chain, aka ETC), which turns oxygen into water. This copper-dependent process releases three energy precursor molecules called adenosine diphosphate (ADP). Once ADP is released, it undergoes a further transformation to create adenosine triphosphate (ATP) at Complex V (also a copper-dependent process), which for all practical purposes should be called Mg-ATP, because that's how the body views it, and uses it. And that's one of the many reasons why magnesium is so important in this quest for optimal energy.

Invariably, in this overall energy-producing process, exhaust is given off, similar to what happens when we start and drive our cars.

When you drive your car, you know that there's exhaust coming out. Similarly, copper is able to run a whole series of enzymes, including ceruloplasmin, that are designed to take the sting out of the oxidants produced by the activation of oxygen. Without ceruloplasmin, these "accidents with oxygen" turn into free radicals that "rust" out our tissues and organs. And please keep in mind, the bulk of all of this activity takes place in our 40 quadrillion (*that's 15 zeroes!*) mitochondria that populate each and every human body. These organelles are the source of 90 percent of the body's energy AND 90 percent of its exhaust! (This will all be explained in more detail in the coming chapters of this book.)

Now you can see why copper is such an important part of mitochondrial function. It is, in fact, of paramount importance. **No or low bioavailable copper inevitably means no or low energy!** Please take a moment and let that reality sink in. Despite the oft repeated phrase that we are "copper toxic," the reality is, for a fact, **just the opposite.** And this bold, counter-cultural statement is backed by extensive scientific research and also supported by thousands of client results.

In summary, even though we are all different, all of our cells are designed to engage in two fundamental actions: create Energy and clear Exhaust. In order to do that, all of our cells rely on a balance of three key minerals (magnesium, copper, and iron), along with ceruloplasmin, to function properly. The fact that you are still struggling with fatigue, but have never heard these concepts before should be an important clue that these principles are true.

All of the above information has been known by scientists for many decades, and has been verified by a great deal of research and countless published scientific studies. I have spent thousands of hours (two to three hours a day, seven days per week for over a decade) pouring through this research to read, reflect, and synthesize what it reveals about these concepts. And yet, these mineral and metabolic truths are all being overlooked, misunderstood, and, worse yet, not being taught to doctors and other health practitioners.

Vitally important discoveries that began in the early 20th century and continue to be made today are not effectively being communicated to those who are trained to guide us in our health decisions. We want to trust our doctors/health practitioners, but unfortunately to no fault of their own, they are not taught this fundamental information about how the cells in our body work. This lack of knowledge in healthcare and across the population leads to the problem of attaining and retaining our vitality and our health, as I explain in the next chapter.

CHAPTER 2

Modern Day Health Solutions That Are Anything But

"We live in a fantasy world, a world of illusion. The great task in life is to find reality."
– Iris Murdoch (1919–1999)

"Nothing is more sad than the death of an illusion."
– Arthur Koestler (1905–1983)

It's often said that the road to hell is paved with good intentions. That sentiment is certainly apt when we consider some of the mainstream lifestyle and medical recommendations from the 20th century that were purportedly dispense to improve our well-being, but on the contrary, proved to be misguided, misleading and detrimental to our health. Broadly speaking, these developments occurred in three key areas: agriculture, gastronomy (the American diet), and medicine. Each has had the detrimental effect of creating our current "Crisis of Mineral Deficiency" by reducing the presence of key minerals, especially copper and magnesium, in our environment, and thus our physiology, while simultaneously increasing iron in our food environment, and subsequently in our bodies' tissues.

What follow are overviews of what has happened in each of these areas since the early 20th century and why they are most responsible for transforming America, and indeed much of the rest of the world, into a sick and chronically tired populace. These next sections provide insights into how we've been misled and misfed.

Agriculture

Thanks to the genius of Pastor Joey Foster (LaPlata, MD), I've learned that *"missing information means missing truth,"* and have adapted that saying to "missing minerals means missing metabolism!" Where this problem really originates is on the farm.

At the beginning of the 20thcentury, America's farmland was a cornucopia of minerals and microbes essential for providing the overall nutrient content of the grains, fruits, vegetables, and livestock that American farmers produce. During that same time, most farmland was owned and managed by local farmers and the crops they produced and harvested were then sold to their local communities.

But then, around the same time as the beginning of today's modern American medical system, everything started to change, leading to the loss of minerals in soil that has been cataloged methodically for the past 90 years (see McCance & Widdowson's "The Composition of Foods," 1930 to 2019). With the advent of modern technologies such as refrigeration, coupled with our growing railway system that made it possible to inexpensively transport food crops across great distances, traditional farming methods soon began to be replaced by commercial farming methods which today have displaced most local farmers with "factory farm" conglomerates whose primary concern is to produce food as cheaply and quickly as possible.

This trend may have been well-intentioned, but it has also proved to be disastrous to our health. Consider refrigeration as one significant example. With its introduction, we lost two-thirds of our exposure to mineral-rich sea salt. Prior to the introduction of refrigeration, foods were packed in sea salt and the American diet was rich in minerals. The advent of the "ice box" played a major role in drastically reducing the mineral content of our food.

But that is far from the only problem. Instead of growing their harvests the way our ancestors did, using only natural fertilizers and annually rotating crops to ensure that cropland remained vitalized and retained its mineral-rich content, modern farming methods rely on a cocktail of manmade chemical fertilizers, pesticides, and other unnatural agents in order to boost production. These chemicals have had a decidedly negative impact on the soil microbes that are key to nutrient uptake by the plants. Most farmers in America, as well as in many other parts of the world, no longer use "rock dust" nor fulvic acid, both of which are well-known means of re-mineralizing the soil. Soil without minerals equals mere dirt, not true cropland teeming with microbial life and vitalizing nutrients.

In addition, today the use of NPK (nitrogen-phosphorus-potassium) is commonly used in crop fertilizers. NPK has known properties that block the uptake of copper by food crops. This fact was well established by Andre Voisin, PhD, in his book *Soil, Grass, Cancer*, originally published in 1959. Voisin was both a farmer and a biochemist who taught biochemistry at the National Veterinary School of France and at the Institute of Tropical Veterinary Medicine in Paris. He believed that simply observing the relationship between farm animals, especially cows, and grass was more valuable than carrying out laboratory experiments. As a result of his observations, he realized that if crop soil and grasses are properly managed and provided with the minerals they require, the animals who live and feed on them would be healthy, as would, in turn, humans who consumed the animal products and crops grown on such soil. In addition, he studied and mapped the elements of the soil and their effects on plants, animals, and humans, and warned against the hidden dangers in modern fertilization practices and the use of toxic chemicals that ignore the delicate balance of trace minerals and nutrients in the soil. Sadly, the findings he published were largely ignored and continue to be disregarded today.

Another problem is the widespread use of antibiotics that are routinely used in commercial farming. These have devastating effects on the mineral status of crop soil and food crops, especially with regard to magnesium and copper. Then, once crops are harvested, more chemical preservatives, wax coatings, and other compounds are added to fruits and vegetables so that they don't spoil as they are shipped across the country and to other lands. Additionally, much of our nation's food supply today comes from other countries where food safety standards are even less stringent than those of commercial factory farms in the United States. As a result, not only are foods today far less nutritious than the food grown by our ancestors, but our cropland is also much more vulnerable because of how depleted of minerals and microbes commercial farming methods have made it. Furthermore, much of today's food is picked before it is ripe so that it can be shipped greater distances without spoilage. It is in this ripening process that the nutrients from the soil (if there) are absorbed by the plant and incorporated into our whole foods.

But perhaps the most serious danger in modern agriculture is the pesticide "Roundup," known chemically as glyphosate. Glyphosate is a true poison and chelates or removes all minerals from the soil, but especially copper. Glyphosate chelates copper down to a pH of 1.0. According to Stephanie Seneff, PhD, one of the world's foremost experts on the dangers to human health caused by glyphosate, that capacity to chelate at low pH means that nothing is capable of stopping glyphosate's chelating action in the soil, plants, animals, and humans (Seneff &Samsel, 2013; 2014; 2015; 2016a [V]; 2016b [VI]; 2017).

In addition, there are sixteen "conserved glycine amino acids" that are essential to make the key copper protein ceruloplasmin. Glyphosate is glycine with a "nitrogen wart." Therefore, Dr. Seneff points out, glyphosate detrimentally affects the inherent production of this key copper protein in our bodies. One of the greatest travesties of our times is that the vast majority of farmers, physicians, and the public at large are completely unaware about this ubiquitous farming chemical's true impact on this critical copper protein, which is the master antioxidant protein for our metabolism.

Besides being sprayed on crops and soil as a weed-killer, glyphosate is now used up to four times each growing season as a desiccant to accelerate the drying out process of wheat, making it easier for farmers to harvest. Based on her research, Dr. Seneff has determined that it is glyphosate residue in wheat and wheat products, not gluten, that is primarily responsible for the large increase in celiac disease and other gastrointestinal disorders attributed to gluten sensitivity. It's also worth noting that, in addition to being bathed with glyphosate, today's modern 18-inch high hybrid wheat is a vastly different, nutritionally-lacking product compared to the Einchorn wheat consumed by our ancestors that stands 48 inches high and is brimming with minerals and vitalizing nutrients.

Although in recent years there has a been a growing trend towards organic farming methods, as well as a rise in the number of Americans who are choosing to support their local farmers by buying locally, either directly from the farmers themselves or at community farmers markets, that still doesn't rectify the problem. For one thing, the soil of organic farms still has a long way to go before it will rival the mineral content of soil from more than a century ago. For another, organic, as well as commercial farmers use fertilizers that contain such compounds as NPK, which limit the ability of plant foods to take in and store copper and magnesium.

The number one nutrient deficiency on the farm is copper deficiency. According to Ben Edwards, MD, there has been an 80 percent loss of copper in crop soil over the past 80 years, and this trend continues. (Based on the pioneering and enduring work of McCance and Widdowson, *The Composition of Foods* published by the Institute for Food Research) That fact alone accounts for most of the reasons why our nation's health is in such a sorry and declining state.

Gastronomy: Iron-"Enriched" Foods and the Low-Fat American Diet

As farming methods began to deteriorate, similar trends began to cross over into the American diet. Beginning in the 1920s, for instance, food processing methods were introduced to "refine" food. Essentially, these so-called refinements stripped out most, if not all, of the nutrients the foods contained. And then, making matters worse, refined sugars were added to processed foods as an inducement to get people to eat them. Few people outside of Meira Fields, PhD and her colleagues at the USDA know that increasing dietary sugar has a decidedly negative effect on copper and magnesium status. Every front has a back, and generations of Americans have suffered from diets centered around processed foods and laden with addictive, mineral-depleting refined sugars.

Then, starting in 1941, matters worsened when inorganic iron filings were added to our food system via enriched wheat flour and grain-based products (Moon, *Iron: The Most Toxic Metal*, 2008). This practice began in the United States, Canada, and Britain, ostensibly to protect against iron-deficiency anemia, a condition that, as you will continue to learn in this book, doesn't actually exist. *(Yes, that's a bold statement, but it is backed by a raft of scientific documentation.)* In

1969, this addition of iron filings was increased by 50 percent based on recommendations by the Food and Drug Administration (FDA). Initially, the FDA sought to triple the amount of added iron. Only after dozens of scientists from around the world testified against this action in Washington, DC, did the FDA acquiesce and only approve a 50 percent increase (Moon, 2008).

Iron is, without question, the metal that ages us (Ashraf et al, 2018). Please re-read that sentence, again... *Iron is the master pro-oxidant element on planet Earth and is the principal element behind what is called oxidative stress.* It's also the trigger for the loss of magnesium that leads to chronic inflammation. It's very important to understand how these two minerals relate to each other. There is a chicken and the egg phenomenon in the body between magnesium deficiency and oxidative stress. Given the known oxidative properties of iron, it stands to reason that, as excess unbound iron rises, magnesium will be lost to that rising oxidative stress. (We're at "Ground Zero" for metabolic dynamics with these reactions and relationships.) Understanding how iron and magnesium relate to one another is key for identifying how to overcome oxidative stress. This is a very important and critical mineral dynamic to understand.

Most of the foods we consume today are woefully lacking in magnesium, and the grain products that comprise an inordinate percentage of the standard American diet are overly loaded with iron. Precisely the opposite of what our ancestors ate and what we need to stay healthy.

Adding insult to iron injury was the adoption of the "low fat" diet that was originally introduced following President Eisenhower's first heart attack in September, 1955 (Keyes, 1955). These dietary recommendations were designed to reduce, even eliminate, cholesterol in the American diet. These guidelines gave rise to the cholesterol myth, one of the biggest medical fallacies still adhered to by many doctors and much of the public today. According to this myth, cholesterol is a risk factor for disease, especially heart attacks, strokes, and other cardiovascular conditions. Because of how cholesterol continues to be demonized in conventional medicine — especially low-density lipoprotein (LDL) cholesterol—cholesterol-lowering drugs, in the form of statins, are today the most widely prescribed class of medications in the United States today. Many doctors are even calling for statins to be administered to pre-teens and teenagers to prevent heart disease. Additionally, for decades, the medical profession has urged us all to avoid eating too much fat and cholesterol-containing foods.

But is cholesterol truly the villain in this story? Most emphatically, "No!" This false narrative was definitively and finally "put to rest" in a recent study by Ravsnkov, Diamond et al, 2016.

Each and every day, our liver produces around 1000 milligrams of cholesterol. Moreover, studies have shown that when people eliminate or restrict their intake of cholesterol-rich foods, liver production of cholesterol increases by as much as an additional 500 mg. Given that the human body is designed to keep itself alive through a continuous repair and adjustment process known as homeostasis, why would it produce so much cholesterol if cholesterol poses a threat to its health?

It doesn't.

The truth is that we would not be alive were it not for cholesterol. It is essential for many of the functions that keep us alive and healthy. Cholesterol is the most important component and structural unit of cell membranes (Zuo H et al, 2015). It maintains the integrity of the cell membrane which encloses and protects the cells themselves. Cholesterol is a vital constituent for a normal functioning nervous system. It plays an important role in the developmental stage and in mature adulthood (Zhang J, Liu Q, 2015) Cholesterol is also needed by our body to manufacture various hormones, and to produce fat-soluble vitamins, steroid hormones, and the bile salts our body requires to absorb fats.

Cholesterol also acts as a natural anti-inflammatory agent. When inflammation is present in the body, cholesterol levels automatically rise as the body attempts to cope with the rising levels of inflammation.

The medical profession has for decades been erroneously attacking cholesterol, one of the most important biomolecules in the human body, while ignoring the fact that iron is one of the most toxic pro-oxidant metals that has been proven, time and again to be at the very epicenter of this our nation's cardiovascular crisis (Sullivan, 1972; Weinberg, 2009; Klevay, 2000). It was iron all along that caused the LDL cholesterol to become "rusty" and lead to the build-up of coronary plaque. What physicians are clearly not taught in medical school is that it requires 11 oxygen molecules to make one cholesterol molecule, nor are they taught that iron oxidizes biomolecules ALL OVER THE BODY!

In effect, cholesterol is a "sink" for excess oxygen, especially when oxidative stress starts rising. Cholesterol's evolution alongside oxygen's appearance on this planet was no accident. Furthermore, cholesterol always rises in the presence of increased oxidative stress (especially when it involves increased hydrogen peroxide, or H_2O_2), which rises as copper becomes bio-unavailable and iron becomes unbound, dominant, and more reactive in our metabolism. All sterols, especially cholesterol, are essential for healthy aerobic metabolism in humans. Their elimination from our foods and our blood, via statins and low-fat dietary restrictions, has only increased our rate of oxidative stress or "rusting."

One of the dire, yet little known, consequences of the low-fat, anti-cholesterol diet is the significant reduction in the intake of retinol, which is the only true form of vitamin A. Retinol, aka pre-formed vitamin A, is a fat-soluble vitamin that is only found in animal-sourced foods, such as liver, oily fish, cheese, butter, heavy cream and egg yolks. Retinol plays an essential role in body growth, immune function, vision and reproductive health. Retinol is essential for the body to maintain homeostasis of copper and it does so through its interactions with the human copper ATPases, ATP7A and ATP7B (Lutsenko et al, 2007). Both ATP7A and ATP7B require retinol to load copper into their copper pumps and to control the production of a network of 12 copper-driven enzymes that regulate and run human metabolism (Hamilton & Lutsenko, 2016).

The person most responsible for the demonization of cholesterol was Ancel Keys. Keys suspected that a fat-rich diet was responsible for heart disease and overall poor health (Keys et al, 1952). To test his hypothesis, he conducted what is known as the Seven Countries Study. The study was so named because it involved studying the diets of populations in Finland, Greece, Japan, Italy, Netherlands, Yugoslavia, and the United States. From this study Keys claimed proof that cholesterol levels were strongly related to heart disease mortality.

Keys' study was highly flawed because, among other things, he buried the findings of 15 other countries that contradicted his findings in the original seven countries. Yet, Keys remained adamant that dietary saturated fats caused elevated cholesterol levels, which in turn caused heart disease. In 1957, the American Heart Association (AHA) joined forces with him (Page et al, 1957. Atherosclerosis and the Fat Content of the Diet. *Circulation* 16:163-178). Soon, AHA spokespersons took to television to warn the American public about the dangers of butter, eggs, bacon, and other saturated fat food sources in relation to heart disease. The US government quickly followed suit, issuing federal guidelines recommending that a low-fat diet be followed in order to prevent heart disease.

It was not long before the high cholesterol/"fat intoxication"/ blocked artery model of heart disease and the proclaimed need for a low-fat diet became accepted as steadfast facts. The belief that this is so still persists today. It was also one of the principal rationales for the creation of the USDA Food Pyramid that occurred in the late 1960s, largely due to the work of Senator George McGovern and his staff, following his appointment by the US Senate to chair the "Select Committee on Nutrition and Human Needs." Influenced by Keys' and the AHA's stance on cholesterol, McGovern's committee proposed that fat and cholesterol consumption be reduced for better heart health. Their doing so led to the creation of the modern USDA Food Pyramid, which in its original form also recommended a high intake of excessively iron-laden grains and other carbohydrates, as well as a low-salt diet. This diet was another incomplete practice that has had devastating effects on our electrolyte balances, and our adrenal glands. which can cause aldosterone levels in the body to rise. Aldosterone is a steroid hormone in the body that is responsible for regulating the balance between salt and other electrolytes. Elevated aldosterone levels are not our friend. Our body is designed for salt and the presence of minerals to run our electrical biochemistry. Too much aldosterone disrupts this essential process of homeostasis.

Because of the faulty "science" upon which its creation was based, today it is widely recognized that the USDA's recommendations for low-fat eating played a significant role in the obesity epidemic that has insidiously gripped America and has exhausted our healthcare system for the last 50 years. Yes, adoption of the "low fat" diet has created a nation of "high fat" citizens.

As an added insult to our health, to attempt to counteract the decline in our health that has resulted from the above developments, we have increasingly been advised to supplement our diet with vitamins and minerals such as synthetic vitamin C (ascorbic acid), vitamin D, calcium, iron, and zinc, all of which further stress the body's mineral status or weaken our immune system. Here again, the end result is a nation that is fatter, sicker, and more tired than ever before in its history. (You will learn the reason why these supplements noted above are detrimental to your health and are causing you to stay tired in Part Two of this book. There, you will also learn of the work of Weston A. Price, DDS, whose research is the cornerstone of nutritional truth regarding what humans should consider and consume as food. His dietary recommendations encompass the Ancestral Diet in its truest form, which I outline and discuss in Chapter 9.)

Modern Medicine

The one consistent finding I've discovered in talking with over 100 doctors and other health care practitioners is that they have never heard, learned about, nor understood the paramount role copper plays in harnessing oxygen and, thereby, protecting our health. That was one of the first comments that Ben Edwards, MD, made in my initial conversations with him: "Morley, I don't recall ever hearing the word 'copper' during my entire classroom or clinical training."

And it's not just copper. There is a total lack of awareness and understanding within the medical community regarding minerals and the essential roles that they play. This is why I affectionately refer to doctors (think MDs) as "M.ineral D.enialists." I am hopeful that this simple book can be viewed as an invitation for doctors – of all faiths and persuasions – to learn aspects of metabolism and energy production that they simply were not taught about in their clinical training. In my opinion, the interplay between copper, ceruloplasmin, iron, magnesium, and oxygen, as well as the countless downstream metabolic processes that they regulate, are among the most important keys to health. They comprise the foundation to our immune system and metabolism, now known as our immunometabolism system. Doctors may talk about the dangers of oxidative stress, but they lack the awareness of what causes it, and therefore are not fully equipped to prevent or to reverse it. Hopefully this book will invite dialogue and inspire further research and understanding.

Despite their eight years or more of formal training that they devote to becoming doctors, medical school students receive virtually no education at all about overall nutrition, let alone mineral metabolism. Case in point: as I write this, this year's graduating class at the University of North Carolina Medical School received a total of only 36 minutes of formal nutrition education during their entire four years of medical school training! How much of such a huge topic can a student learn, and then apply competently after receiving only 36 minutes of instruction?

And beyond these basics, there is also a lack of awareness about "energy deficiency" in modern medicine. There is no yardstick for measuring a patient's energy level or ATP status. There is no understanding of how ATP is actually made within the countless mitochondria that reside in our tissues, nor of the scale of how many mitochondria are needed to support optimal human metabolism. And while there is a general acceptance of the term "mitochondrial dysfunction" by most doctors, modern medicine remains blind to the fact that said dysfunction is largely, if not solely, due to mineral deficiencies and imbalances.

How can that be?

The answer lies with the transformation of modern medicine that began over a century ago. At the dawn of the 20th century, at least 25 percent of all health care providers in the US practiced some form of medicine that, at least to some extent, emphasized the importance of diet and nutrition as primary preventive and therapeutic treatments. At the same time, however, medical schools had no uniform standards of education.

Recognizing this fact, members of the Carnegie Foundation—named after its founder, Andrew Carnegie, one of the wealthiest men in the world at that time—decided that improving medical education should be a primary goal of its philanthropic mission. To this end, Henry Pritchett, the Foundation's head, hired Abraham Flexner to assess the overall status of medical education in both the United States and Canada.

According to Thomas P. Duffy, MD, Pritchett and his associates, "perceived the problem of medical education as a problem of education and believed a professional educator, like Flexner, was better qualified to address this dimension of the problem. They also had preconceived ideas concerning what changes needed to be made in medical schools to allow these ideas to be introduced...An unflattering but not necessarily inaccurate description for Flexner's assignment was that he was to be the hatchet man in sweeping clean the medical system of substandard medical schools that were flooding the nation with poorly trained physicians." (Duffy, Thomas P, 2011-Sep, The Flexner Report-100 Years On. *Yale J Biol Med*; 84(3): 269–276.)

In 1910, Flexner achieved Pritchett's aims with his book-length publication, *Medical Education in the United States and Canada*, commonly referred to today as The Flexner Report. As a direct result of The Flexner Report, many US and Canadian medical schools were forced to close, and most of the remaining schools underwent a "reformation" in order to conform to the model Flexner advocated.

While this resulted in many needed improvements in the medical education offered by the remaining schools, it also resulted in a strong bias in favor of a model that led to the narrow symptom-centered, drug-based treatment regimens practiced by doctors today. Lost among the reorganization and the revamping were whole-patient care and other treatment options, like diet and nutrition. As Dr. Duffy states, "There was maldevelopment in the structure of medical education in America in the aftermath of the Flexner Report... Flexner's corpus [his report] was all nerves without the life blood of caring." It was also devoid of any understanding of the importance minerals play in our metabolism and mitochondria-derived energy production, let alone the root cause of fatigue and disease.

During this same time, the use of petrochemicals, which are chemicals derived from petroleum, in the preparation and manufacture of pharmaceutical drugs was also underway. For example, the petroleum compound phenol was used as a preparatory substance to manufacture aspirin, and petroleum resins in general played a role in drug purification procedures. As a side note, an important fact that is often overlooked or unknown by most doctors is that polyphenol oxidase is one of the most important copper-dependent enzymes of the over 500 enzymes in our livers. Therefore, it stands to reason that copper as a cofactor to this enzyme must be key to metabolizing all of these phenol-containing pharmaceutical drugs. Petrochemicals are still widely used in the manufacture of most pharmaceutical drugs today.

The dominance of the pharmaceutical drug model in what passes for "healthcare" today has had and continues to have serious negative health consequences. The full scope of these consequences was highlighted in a report by Donald W. Light, PhD, published by Harvard University's Edmond J. Safra Center for Ethics. In that report, Light states, "Few people know that new prescription drugs have a one in five chance of causing serious reactions after they have been approved. That is why expert physicians recommend not taking new drugs for at least five years unless patients have first tried better-established options, and have the need to do so.

"Few know that systematic reviews of hospital charts found that even properly prescribed drugs (aside from mis-prescribing, overdosing, or self-prescribing) cause about 1.9 million hospitalizations a year. Another 840,000 hospitalized patients are given drugs that cause serious adverse reactions for a total of 2.74 million serious adverse drug reactions. About 128,000 people die from drugs prescribed to them. This makes prescription drugs a major health risk, ranking 4th with stroke as a leading cause of death. The European Commission estimates that adverse reactions from prescription drugs cause 200,000 deaths; so together, about 328,000 patients in the US and Europe die from prescription drugs each year. The FDA does not acknowledge these facts and instead gathers a small fraction of the cases." (Light, Donald W. 2014-June 27,. *New Prescription Drugs: A Major Health Risk With Few Offsetting Advantages*). https://ethics.harvard.edu/blog/new-prescription-drugs-major-health-risk-few-offsettingadvantages

Pharmaceutical drugs pose other serious problems, as well. Many pharmaceutical drugs contain some form of fluoride, which inactivates magnesium and prevents magnesium uptake. In addition, many drugs directly deplete magnesium and copper. These include diet pills, diuretics, many high blood pressure medications, various antibiotics and antifungal drugs, anticancer drugs such as cisplatin, acid blockers and antacids, statins and other cholesterol-lowering drugs, and oral contraceptives. The United States consumes more pharmaceutical drugs per capita—both prescription and over-the-counter—than any other country in the world. With terrible result, I might add. An increasing array of pharmaceutical drugs are now known to cause devastating effects on mineral status in the human body. This is a fact proven over and over again in the medical literature, yet still ignored, or generally unknown by most MDs. However, there are always exceptions like one of my personal heroes, Mildred S. Seelig, MD, MPH. She was originally a drug researcher and switched to becoming a magnesium zealot when she realized that most pharmaceutical drugs caused magnesium loss.

And that's far from the only harm modern medicine is causing. Consider these facts:

- CIPRO and most other antibiotics don't just wipe out "good bacteria" along with the "bad", they are also very hard on copper status resulting in connective tissue disorders.
- Benzodiazepines ("benzos"), a widely prescribed class of drugs, are most destructive to copper status in the brain.
- Various medical procedures and recommendations are also known to block mineral uptake. For example, copper deficiency is a known and recognized side-effect of bariatric surgery and total parenteral nutrition. Zinc supplementation reduces copper uptake in the gut. Chelation therapies bind to copper in the bloodstream, forming a compound that ushers it out of the body.

- Most pharmaceutical drugs also contain iron oxides that further contribute to the iron load that is already being poorly managed by the body for the many reasons already cited. This additional iron only adds to the oxidation/inflammation occurring at the cellular level due to mineral deficiencies, coupled with a lack of ceruloplasmin.

There is also a faulty belief by doctors and scientists in "gene defects," when there is increasing evidence and proof that a weakening bioenergetic field changes the frequency of the tissue that affects all of metabolism, not the least of which are the nucleus of the cell, as well as the mitochondrial DNA that are directly affected by a loss of energy production. Furthermore, there are 16 times more defects in the mitochondrial DNA which directly affects the cell's capacity to produce healthy mitochondria and thereby produce optimal levels of energy. Proper mineral balance is essential for preventing the oxidative stress that is known to cause these genetic changes, and prevent their correction by a network of repair enzymes which require minerals for their activation. The good news is, the body can correct itself if, and when, balanced mineralization is reestablished.

But the ultimate failure of contemporary diagnostic medicine is its abject blind spot about how iron status is best measured in the body. Iron in the tissue can be up to 10 time greater than iron in the blood. (Killilea & Ames, 2004). Yes, there is a notable difference in iron status between tissue and blood. That is a critical factor to understand. The focus in what passes for iron research at present is on the "Labile Iron Pool" (note: "labile" does not mean "free," *it means "reactive"*). If only doctors had been/were more completely trained in what this really represents in terms of the origin of reactive oxygen species (ROS) and oxidative stress inside the mitochondria and the cells. We will learn more about these critical dynamics in Chapter 4.

Nor is there any consideration given to, nor understanding about, the importance of the body's iron reticuloendothelial system (RES) that is intended to re-cycle iron on a daily basis (I refer to RES as the "REcycling System"). Due to the vacuous presence of bioavailable copper, iron ends up getting "sequestered" (stuck) and "stored" in what are known as recycling macrophages (the "Pac-Men" of the body). Based on the pioneering research of Nancy Andrews, MD, PhD (Duke), Rebecca King, MD (Mayo Clinic) and Marianne Wessling-Resnick, PhD (Harvard), this dysfunction in the daily iron recycling program is now theorized to be the metabolic origin for over 100 autoimmune conditions that have been escalating during the last 40 years. The similar spiral of malabsorption syndromes, such as small intestinal bacterial overgrowth (SIBO), leaky gut, Crohn's disease, and colitis that have occurred during the same time period are all caused by excessively high iron levels in the intestinal cells, called enterocytes, that disable proper mineral and energy metabolism. Iron that does not get properly "absorbed"—meaning, released into the blood—festers in the gut tissues, causing iron-induced oxidative stress.

Furthermore, doctors do not understand that excess iron causes copper to become less bioavailable and functional. (Ha, Collins, et al, 2017) That is the real issue underlying what doctors erroneously diagnose as "anemia," and invariably leads to a recommendation of increasing iron uptake through foods, oral supplements and/or intravenous iron transfusions. This anemia dynamic is not "iron deficiency," but is more accurately called "iron dysfunction" that leads to anemia of chronic inflammation (DeDomenico et al, 2008) The REAL issue is a lack of bioavailable copper, not a lack of iron, because copper is essential to activate ferroportin, the only known exporter of iron from cells into the blood. The protein ferroportin and its mechanisms for iron egress requires ferroxidase activity that is only derived from multi-copper oxidase enzymes.

Finally, the switch to measuring iron status via hemoglobin, which was the norm from 1860 until 1972 (Jacobs et al, 1972), to measuring serum (blood) ferritin levels is another major disruption to properly understanding the dynamic between copper and iron. Ferritin, the known iron storage protein, is meant to be inside cells, NOT outside cells -- in the blood. Ferritin is only found in the blood when there is rising inflammation in the tissue, by which time a patient's health status has already been seriously disrupted. That basic fact is not taught properly and completely to doctors, which is leading to an alarming increase in recommendations for iron supplementation. What may come as a surprise is that ferritin in the blood is an "empty shotgun shell," (Worwood, Jacobs et al, 1976; Kell & Pretorius, 2010) and the serum ferritin has very little, if any, iron. Please note, the iron has already been discharged into the organ(s), usually the lysosomes of the liver cells, prior to the secretion of the ferritin into the blood, and the iron that remains accumulates, and then goes on to cause chronic inflammation in that organ.

Given all of the above, it's no wonder that we as a nation, and as a world population for that matter, are excessively sick and exceedingly tired, and that modern medicine has such an incomplete understanding of these KEY mineral/metal dynamics, especially when it comes to improving our health and energy levels.

It's time for all of us to get off this "fast track" to inflammation and recognize that so much of what we have been told about health and how to achieve and maintain it is incomplete and myth-guided. Thus, the premise for my notion that we have been "misled and misfed." In order to reverse this trend, we need to move away from these untruths and myth-truths and replace them with proven scientific facts. Let's start our deep dive towards doing so by exploring how our body really makes energy, which happens to be the focus of the next chapter.

How Your Body Makes Energy– There's More to This Story Than Most Doctors Know

"Life is the interplay between structure and energy, yet the role of energy deficiency in human disease has been poorly explored by modern medicine."
– Douglas C. Wallace, PhD (2005), founder of the field of human mitochondrial DNA (mtDNA) genetics

"Only by understanding the wisdom of the body shall we attain the mystery of disease and pain that will enable us to relieve the burden of people."
– Walter Bradford Cannon, MD (1871–1945)

Has this ever happened to you?

Suffering from persistent fatigue, you go to your doctor, hoping for help. He or she orders a series of blood tests for you and when the results come back you are told, "Everything looks normal." Then, instead of having an actual solution to offer you, your doctor leaves you with some pat advice: Be sure to exercise, eat healthy, and get more sleep. All without telling you how to achieve any of this. And, if you're really unlucky, you may be advised to take an iron supplement.

Sadly, the above scenario is quite common in America today. Fatigue continues to be the number one health complaint that doctors hear from their patients, yet the doctors remain clueless about how to help them. Their pat advice doesn't cut it and eventually their patients resign themselves to "just having to live with" being tired all the time.

The reason why this abysmal situation exists is because most doctors don't have a clue about the vital factors that must be addressed to create and maintain abundant levels of energy in the body. In this chapter, I am going to tell you what they were not taught. (Or, if they do know it, they ignore it because it does not fit in with the drug-based, symptom management medical paradigm they insist on remaining stuck within even though, if they are honest with themselves, they would admit how often that paradigm is failing their patients.)

To understand why you are so tired so often, you have to know how your body produces energy and what it needs in order to do so. Then, in order to banish your fatigue, you have to ensure that those needs are met. Happily, none of this is rocket science, and the energy solution you are seeking is something you can provide yourself on your own.

Let me explain.

The Keys To Having More Energy

Here are the essential keys, or factors, you need to know about and understand when it comes to having more energy: the "activation" of both hydrogen and oxygen to make water, the recycling of ADP and ATP inside our mitochondria (our cells' "powergrid"), and the dynamic interaction of copper, iron, magnesium, and ceruloplasmin to make it all possible.

Despite all of the complex mechanisms involved in the body's production of energy, they can all accurately be distilled down into a three-step process. 1. Hydrogen and oxygen combine to make water. 2. Once produced, water enables the release of copper-dependent ADP (adenosine diphosphate) that get transformed into Mg-ATP (adenosine triphosphate) in another copper-dependent step in the mitochondria. 3. And—an extremely crucial key that most doctors either do not know or fully understand—copper, via ceruloplasmin, supports these metabolic processes and prevents iron from causing the oxidants thrown off by this process from rusting out the body's tissues and organs. (Remember, as you learned in Chapter 1, during this overall process, as energy is produced, exhaust is also produced in the form of oxidants—or "accidents with oxidants," as I call them. This is very similar to what happens when we run our cars.)

Scientists estimate that we produce the equivalent of our body weight in ATP each and every day, and expend one billion ATP for each beat of our heart. Our need for energy and for Mg-ATP is relentless.

Cellular Respiration: The above three-step process of energy production occurs through what is known as cellular respiration. Here is an overview of what happens as the process of cellular respiration unfolds.

You learned in school that when your breathe, you take in oxygen when you inhale, and release carbon dioxide when you exhale. Both of these gases—oxygen (O_2) and carbon dioxide (CO_2)—are used by your body's cells during cellular respiration to break down molecules to produce energy. The main molecules that are broken down in this process are hydrocarbons, called sugar (glucose) and fat (lipids) molecules that are obtained from the foods we eat. What happens during cellular respiration is that the oxygen we breathe in and the glucose and/or fat from our diet are transformed into carbon dioxide, water, and energy in the form of ATP. During this process, the atoms within the molecules are rearranged, but nothing new is created, and nothing is destroyed. In physics, the fact that energy can neither be created nor destroyed is known as the law of conservation of energy, which was first proposed and scientifically tested by the French philosopher, scientist, and mathematician Émilie du Châtelet (1706–1749).

The most efficient form of cellular respiration is aerobic respiration, meaning respiration that requires the presence of oxygen. Plants, animals, and humans all utilize aerobic cellular respiration. The only difference is that plants obtain the molecules they need for it from photosynthesis, whereas animals and humans obtain them from the foods they eat. The overall chemical equation for cellular respiration in animals and humans is $C_6H_{12}O_6$ (glucose) + 6 O_2 (6 oxygen atoms) → 6 CO_2 (6 carbon dioxide atoms) + 6 H_2O (6 water atoms) + 36 ATP (36 atoms of adenosine triphosphate). And depending on the type of fat being consumed, the number of energy molecules can be anywhere from 130 to 140 ATP per unit of fat. This is why fat is such an important part of our diet. It is a pivotal part of our energy generating process. (Btw, please compare this energy equation above to the chemical equation for photosynthesis: $6CO_2$ + 6 H_2O + sunlight → $C_6H_{12}O_6$ + $6O_2$ – same components, but different order).

In the animal and human chemical equation, glucose/fat and oxygen act as reactants, meaning they are the precursor substances that are transformed into the end products of carbon dioxide, water, and ATP.

The equation itself does not tell the whole story of cellular respiration, though, reducing as it does three processes into a single one. As I mentioned above, energy production in the body actually occurs in three stages, as does cellular respiration. Its stages and metabolic pathways are glycolysis; the Krebs, or TCA (citric acid cycle); and the ETC (electron transport chain) and what is known as oxidative phosphorylation.

Glycolysis is a term derived from the Greek language and literally translates as "sugar splitting." It occurs within the fluid inside your cells known as cytosol, also referred to as the intercellular matrix. This step occurs without oxygen, meaning it is anaerobic.

Glycolysis begins when a glucose molecule is split into two molecules of pyruvate. This split occurs due to the energy of ATP, specifically two ATP molecules. This is known as the energy investment phase. Two ATP molecules are consumed to eventually make two molecules of pyruvate, while also generating two molecules of ATP. This is known as the energy return phase, since, though the process started with two molecules of ATP, an energy return of four ATP molecules occurs, resulting in a net yield of two new ATP molecules. In this process, two molecules of NADH (nicotinamide adenine dinucleotide) are also produced. The pyruvate will then go onto the Krebs cycle, while the NADH will go onto the ETC (electron transport chain), both actions taking place within the mitochondria.

Referring back to the chemical equation for cellular respiration, once the process of glycolysis is complete, while glucose has been used, oxygen, carbon dioxide and water have not been used, and only two molecules of the necessary 36 have been produced, leaving 34 more still to be produced.

The next stage occurs as the Krebs, or TCA (citric acid cycle). You may have learned about the Krebs cycle in school. It was discovered by and is named after Hans Adolf Krebs, MD, PhD (Aug 25, 1900 - Nov 22, 1981), a pioneering physician, biologist, and biochemist who received a Nobel Prize in 1953 from his discoveries regarding cellular energy production.

In this stage of cellular respiration, the pyruvate molecules created during the glycolysis stage are oxidized inside the mitochondrial matrix to produce a compound called acetyl-coenzyme A (acetyl-CoA) during what is known as the prep stage. The Krebs cycle is then initiated, which causes acetyl-CoA to become oxidized to two carbon dioxide (CO_2) molecules and two more molecules of NADH. Then, through a series of additional steps, four more molecules of CO_2 are produced, as well as six additional NADH molecules, two molecules of FADH2 (flavin adenine dinucleotide, a redox-active coenzyme), and two more molecules of ATP. All of this happening in nanoseconds, day and night.

Returning to the cellular respiration equation, by the end of the Krebs cycle, glucose has been completely broken down. Oxygen and water still have not been produced, however, but all six CO_2 molecules have, as well as two additional ATP molecules. What remains is for the 10 NADH and two FADH2 molecules to enter the ETC (electron transport chain). Both NADH and FADH2 are known as high-energy electron carriers that are key to the actions of the ETC.

The electron transport chain (ETC) is a series of enzymes embedded in the inner membrane of the mitochondria. As electrons are passed along from one respiratory enzyme to the next, energy is harnessed to produce ATP. This is what occurs as the electrons within NADH and FADH2 enter the final step of the ETC through a process called oxidative phosphorylation. In layperson's terms, what happens is that, as the high-energy electrons within NADH and FADH2 interact with the enzymes within the mitochondrial membrane, the enzymes transport the electrons down the line of the ETC, and hydrogen protons are pumped to the outer compartment of the mitochondria.

At this stage, oxygen enters the equation, grabbing the hydrogen protons to produce two molecules of water. At the same time, an additional 32 molecules of ATP are produced by a key respiratory protein/enzyme called ATP synthase through the movement of ions across a membrane down to their electrochemical gradient. This process is known as chemiosmosis, and earned Peter D. Mitchell, PhD, FRS a Nobel Prize in 1978 for his genius to sort this out.

This electron transfer is driven by the chemical energy of oxygen interacting with the two hydrogen protons to form water. At the completion of this process, the entire cycle of cellular respiration is complete, resulting in a net production of 36 ATP molecules.

To summarize this entire process, mitochondria convert chemical energy from glucose and fat in the cell into energy (ATP) that is made usable to the cell, with the final process occurring inside the mitochondria, within the respiratory complexes I-IV of the ETC, ending with Complex V, called oxidative phosphorylation. The end result is the generation of adenosine triphosphate (ATP), which serves as the "fuel" of the cells. It is worth noting that this last complex, ATP synthase, is a nano-rotor spinning at 9,000 rpms and produce 3 ATP with each full rotation. Therefore, 27,000 ATP are produced by each ATP synthase each and every minute. Most importantly, this final complex requires the presence of BOTH magnesium and copper!

This process is repeated continuously within the cells of our body every moment of our entire lives. How efficiently it is performed determines how much energy we will have. Alas, for most people, it is not being performed efficiently at all, and the reasons why will soon be made clear. First, though, let's take a closer look at the cells' mitochondria.

Remarkable Mitochondria

Given how most of the cellular respiration cycle occurs inside the mitochondria, you can understand why mitochondria are often referred to as the cells' "energy factories" or "powerhouses."

Here are some interesting facts about mitochondria: They are constantly dividing and bonding together, and are linked together in ever-changing networks. Truth be known, there are more like "power grids" than "energy factories" (Glancy B. 2015; 2019) They have their own set of DNA, which is similar to bacteria DNA.

Though you received half of your human DNA from your father and half from your mother, all of your mitochondrial DNA (mtDNA) came from your mother. For this reason, mtDNA is now used as an effective method for tracing and analyzing ancestral genetic lines. The scientist who figured these concepts out is Douglas Wallace, PhD, who provided the opening quotation to this chapter.

In many respects, we might consider mitochondria to be "cells within cells," since all functions in the body begin at the cellular level, and cells cannot function properly without the mitochondria the cells contain. (The only exceptions are red blood cells, which contain no mitochondria and make their energy anaerobically to perform their functions.) Similarly, just as the health of the cells depends on what we supply our bodies (food, water, oxygen, etc.), so too are mitochondria dependent on their host cells to provide them with the "food" (glucose/fat) and oxygen they require to perform their tasks.

Because mitochondria are able to divide on their own, they are able to increase their number in each cell to meet the energy demands of each type of cell they are found in. Heart muscle cells have the highest energy demand of all cells in the body because the constantly beating heart works harder than any other organ in your body. Therefore, it is not surprising that approximately 40 percent of the cytoplasm in heart muscle cells is taken up by mitochondria (roughly 10,000 mitochondria in each heart muscle cell). Liver cells also have a high energy demand, and between 20 and 25 percent of liver cell cytoplasm space is taken up by mitochondria (~2,000 mitochondria per cell). By contrast, the tissue of the biceps muscle only has about 500 mitochondria per cell, since its energy demands are considerably less.

In addition to supplying energy, mitochondria perform a number of other vital functions. One of these functions is determining when cells will recycle via autophagy or die— either via ordinary cell death, known as necrosis, or programmed cell death, known as apoptosis. Mitochondria initiate apoptosis by releasing a chemical known as cytochrome c, which, in turn, activates caspase, one of the primary lysosomal enzymes that are designed to destroy aging cells during the process of apoptosis. Mitochondria's role in apoptosis is particularly important because apoptosis prevents aging or damaged cells from becoming cancer cells. Impaired mitochondrial function prevents apoptosis from happening, which is why cancer is today increasingly recognized as being due to mitochondrial dysfunction.

In addition, mitochondria play a role in determining which eggs (ovum) in women are released during ovulation, and which are destroyed by apoptosis, as part of a process known as atresia. During atresia, scientists believe that within the ovum the mitochondria and the nucleus of the cell in which mitochondria reside are screened for biocompatibility. If incompatibility exists, the mitochondria initiates apoptosis. What is important to understand is that each egg cell can have as many as 600,000 mitochondria. Therein lies the energy for the start of new life!

Another important role performed by mitochondria has to do with the storage and regulation of calcium. Calcium plays many important functions in the body and is vital for a number of cellular processes, including cellular metabolism. The cells regulate calcium very closely, however, to prevent unchecked calcium buildup. Mitochondria guide this process by quickly absorbing calcium ions when they enter cells and storing them until they are needed.

Mitochondria are also capable of helping the body generate heat, a process known as thermogenesis. The most common form of thermogenesis you may be familiar with is shivering when you are cold. Our bodies shiver to keep us warm.

Heat can also be produced by our bodies in other ways, including using brown fat tissues, also known as BAT (brown adipose tissue). When this happens, the mitochondria are intimately involved, uncoupling proteins to transport protons within brown fat tissues to trigger a form of non-shivering thermogenesis. And it is useful to know that what makes BAT "brown," is a high concentration of mitochondria in those key fat metabolizing cells.

Impaired Mitochondrial Function And Illness: Because of how essential mitochondria are for supplying our body with energy, along with its other vital functions, it should be obvious that keeping mitochondria healthy is of paramount importance. If mitochondria become damaged or otherwise impaired and are unable function properly, our body will start to lose the energy it needs and the stage will be set for a wide range of medical problems to take hold. Again, as Dr. Wallace notes, it is "energy deficiency" that triggers the untold oxidative stress that precedes all symptoms of chronic conditions. Not some, *ALL*.

This brings me back to the point I keep making about how important it is for our bodies to not only be able to create energy, but also to be able to "clear exhaust," meaning the reactive oxygen species (ROS) waste products, including free radicals, that are also produced during the process of cellular respiration. Mitochondrial DNA are far more susceptible to free radical and ROS damage than human DNA in the cell nucleus. In addition, mitochondria also lack many of the various protective mechanisms that help maintain the health and stability of the cell nucleus. In addition, since the ROS that is created during the creation of ATP occurs so near to the mitochondria, mtDNA is up to sixteen times more likely to be damaged by ROS than nuclear DNA (Yakes et al, 1997; Chatterjee et al, 2006; Kawalska et al, 2020), and therefore are also much more likely to experience unhealthy mutations, and at a much faster rate than nuclear DNA might mutate. When mitochondria no longer function properly, more ROS are produced, causing more mitochondria to mutate and be damaged even further.

Mitochondrial mutations and mitochondrial dysfunctions in general are considered (erroneously, as I explain later in this chapter) to be primary causes of the diseases that affect areas of the body that have the highest energy demands, such as the heart, brain, central nervous system, muscles, the liver, the kidneys, the gastrointestinal tract, and the eyes. When mitochondria stop functioning properly, the cells they are in become energy-starved and harbingers of oxidative stress. Either the oxygen gets "activated" cleanly and completely by complex IV to make water to release ATP or this oxygen gets "rusty" and becomes oxidative stress (aka ROS). It is an either/or function that is not fully understood in practitioner circles.

The symptoms that can result from this lack of cellular energy can vary greatly, depending on the type of cell that is so affected. Typically, cells in the areas of the body that need the most energy are most greatly affected by damaged and/or mutated mitochondria. The brain and central nervous system (CNS) are two such areas, which is why people suffering from Alzheimer's disease, Parkinson's disease, Multiple Sclerosis, and other conditions of the brain and CNS usually have a much higher number of damaged mitochondria and/or a greater rate of mitochondrial mutation compared to healthy people. The same is true of people with heart disease, cancer, and various other conditions. Again, it is worth noting that some regions of the brain have as many as two million mitochondria per neuron (nerve cells). This begins to bring new understanding to what the scale of "energy deficiency" might actually be across our body.

Mitochondrial damage and mutation is also a primary cause of premature aging. Though it is natural for some degree of damage and mutation to occur in mitochondria as we age, accelerated rates of either are known to correspondingly accelerate the aging process, as well as cause premature death. This fact was first observed by Denham Harman, PhD, MD (February 14, 1916 – November 25, 2014), the father of what is known as the "free radical theory of aging," which he first proposed in 1956 in his scientific paper published in the *Journal of Gerontology. (Harman, D., 1956, Aging: a theory based on free radical and radiation chemistry. J Gerontology 11(3): 298–300).* It is worth noting that that Dr. Harman updated and revised his theories in 1972 and about the time of his 90th birthday, he further revised his theories in 2006/

The Rest and Most Important Part of The Story

Everything you have read so far in this chapter is well known by doctors and other health practitioners. Or at least it should be.

The problem, though, is that for the most part that is as far as their knowledge goes when it comes to a discussion of energy. They may be able to discuss ATP, the mitochondria, and the process of cellular respiration with you, but what they likely cannot tell you is how to ensure that your body produces energy most effectively and efficiently. They can't tell you that because they don't know the answer to this most basic, yet most important, question.

Why?

Because they have never been taught it.

Sad though this fact is, it's not surprising, since there is a complete lack of awareness of "energy deficiency" in modern medicine. As a result, doctors have no yardstick for measuring a patient's energy level or ATP status. Nor do they have an understanding of how ATP is actually made within the mitochondria, nor of the scale of how many mitochondria are needed to support human life. (Current estimates put this number at 40 quadrillion!) While there may be acceptance of the term "mitochondrial dysfunction" among doctors, modern medicine remains blind to the fact that said dysfunction is largely, if not solely, due to mineral deficiencies. That is the heart of the problem and explains why so few doctors ever succeed in helping their patients "[Cu]re their fatigue" by producing more energy.

More to the point, what doctors don't know is how and why two minerals and one protein are so essential for the proper production of ample energy in the body—indeed, energy production is wholly dependent upon them– and how the entire process of energy production is thwarted by one other mineral when it becomes unbound and excessively builds up in the body.

The two essential minerals for energy production that I am referring to are, first and foremost, copper, and, secondarily, magnesium, and the protein is ceruloplasmin. And iron, which will be discussed in much more detail in Chapter 4, is the mineral that can significantly muck up the production of energy if there is too much of it and it becomes unbound. Which is precisely what has happened in the bodies of everyone who are chronically fatigued and suffering from chronic conditions.

Before I explain the crucial roles copper, magnesium, and ceruloplasmin play in energy production, let's first take a closer general look at each of them.

Copper: Copper is an essential trace mineral. And by essential, I mean absolutely vital. Without enough bioavailable copper your body simply cannot produce all of the energy it needs, and you cannot stay healthy. Copper plays crucial roles in the energy production cycle discussed above. It is required for optimal enzyme activity and the transfer of electrons in the cell, and is an integral part of the 5-part mitochondria's respiratory chain that produces our Mg-ATP.

Specifically, copper is what enables electrons to be transported along the membrane of the mitochondria because of how it aids the pivotal enzyme known as cytochrome-c oxidase (Complex IV) to accept electrons and H+ atoms. Copper is also necessary for generating cytochrome-C oxidase. Complex IV is the final electron acceptor in the cycle of energy production and passes electrons to molecular oxygen. The electrons and oxygen then bind with hydrogen (H+) atoms to produce water and release ATP. Because copper is so essential for proper energy production, it plays many other important roles in the body, including helping to maintain the health of the liver. This is not surprising, since it is in the liver that some of the highest concentrations of copper are found. Your liver is one of your body's most important organs, and also one of the most overworked, being responsible for carrying out more than 500 vital functions, all of which are directly or indirectly dependent on the liver's copper stores and copper-dependent enzymes.

Because of how bioavailable copper helps protect against oxidative stress, copper also helps protect the thyroid gland, as well as all other organs and tissues in the body, from becoming damaged or impaired by ROS and oxidants ("accidents with oxygen"). Copper deficiency can result in thyroiditis, an inflammatory condition in which the thyroid gland becomes injured. Lack of copper can, in particular, cause an increase in superoxide, hydrogen peroxide, and other damaging oxidative molecules. Moreover, without copper, the body's glutathione system cannot function optimally. Glutathione is one of the body's important intracellular antioxidants. Copper is essential for the function of superoxide dismutase (SOD) which regulates antioxidant clean up during the production of thyroid hormones.

Copper also plays vital roles in the immune system's first line of defense against infection. One way that it does that is by aiding in hematopoiesis, the medical term for the formation of heme and blood cells, including red blood cells (RBCs). It is a well known fact that RBCs transport oxygen from the lungs to the cells and carry carbon dioxide back to the lungs, where it is discharged through exhalation. What is less well known is that red blood cells also play a role in the body's innate immune system. Specifically, RBCs have the ability to gather up infectious pathogens and deliver them to immune cells in the spleen, where the pathogens are then destroyed.

The loss or lack of bioavailable copper leads to impairment of the hematopoiesis process, and thus a reduction in the number of red blood cells. Though the connection between copper deficiency and hematopoiesis problems is clearly established in the medical literature, it continues to be overlooked by physicians, who instead tell patients suffering with reduced levels of, or unhealthy, red blood cells, that they have anemia due to a lack of iron. Nothing could be further from the truth. *It is the lack of bioavailable copper that is the problem that needs to be addressed!* (Ames BN, Atamna H, Killilea DK, 2005-Aug, "Mineral and Vitamin Deficiencies Can Accelerate the Mitochondrial Decay of Aging" *Mol Aspects of Medicine* 26(4-5): 363-378 doi:10.1016/j.mam.2005.07.007)

Copper is also vitally important for the production of neutrophils, a primary type of white blood cells. Neutrophils, which are produced in bone marrow, serve as a major defense against infections. They destroy harmful bacteria, as well as various viruses in the blood. Without bioavailable copper within their cells, neutrophils cannot perform these important tasks efficiently because copper deficiency causes them to weaken as they attempt to attack and destroy infectious microorganisms. In addition, copper deficiency can result is reduced numbers of neutrophils, just as it can with red blood cells. This condition is called neutropenia, and is more common that many physicians realize (Percival SS, 1995; Lazarcheck J, 2012; Harless W, 2006).

Although researchers are still trying to more fully understand the mechanisms that cause copper deficiencies to result in neutropenia, it is certain that the role that copper plays in the production of ATP is definitely involved. ATP is crucial for cells such as neutrophils, which have a very high demand for energy. Reduced ATP production due to a lack of copper causes a disruption in the ability of neutrophils to function and to be produced in adequate numbers.

In addition to the above roles, copper is also necessary for the healthy formation of bone, collagen, and connective tissue, and the prevention of certain genetic disorders. Now you understand why I maintain that copper is absolutely crucial for our health, and why I consider physicians who fail to address copper deficiency to be guilty of mineral malpractice. For those that have any doubt about the reach and importance of copper enzymes, you will be well advised to spend time with Heather S. Comstra, et al, 2017-May 29, "The Interactome of the Copper Transporter ATP7A belongs to a network of neurodevelopmental and neurodegeneration factors" *eLife* 6:e24722. We have, indeed, been misled and misfed.

Magnesium: *"Without enough magnesium, cells simply don't work."* This quote by Lawrence M. Resnick, MD, former Professor of Medicine at Weill Cornell Medical School, sums up all you need to know to understand why it is so important that you daily obtain all of the magnesium your body needs. If you suffer from fatigue, you can be sure you also suffer from magnesium deficiency.

For the past four decades, an average of 2,000 scientific studies per year about the health benefits of magnesium have been published in medical journals around the globe. Sadly, for the most part, these studies continue to go unnoticed by the medical community. One such study, published in 2012, detected magnesium binding sites on 3,751 human proteins. This finding proved that magnesium's role in maintaining health and preventing disease is far greater than previously thought. (Piovesan D, et al. 3,751 Magnesium binding sites have been detected on human protein. *BMC Bioinformatics*. 2012; 13 Suppl 14:S10 Epub 2012 Sep 7. PMID: 23095498.) This study presents a vastly different picture of magnesium's role than the oft-quoted reference that "magnesium is important to some 300 enzymes."

Magnesium, primarily acting within our cells, is responsible for the proper functioning of many of the body's metabolic processes. It aids these functions by activating numerous metabolic pathways in the body, including those responsible for protein, carbohydrate, and fat metabolism. Magnesium also plays a vital role in energy metabolism because it is essential for key steps of anaerobic glycolysis and the Krebs cycle, as well as the stabilization of ATP. Magnesium is essential for the production and storage of energy inside each of our 100 trillion cells. That's a lot of ATP, and that's a lot of magnesium, too. An important way of understanding the significance of this activity is, as noted before, that we generate our body weight in Mg-ATP each and every day. And given the magnitude of this daily ATP production, it makes the lack of a clinical "energy yardstick" all the more surreal and significant.

Magnesium is also the essential nutrient for muscles, playing a vital role in their proper functioning and their relaxation, so they can be ready for the next contraction. Without magnesium, there would be no regulation of movement, and our muscles could not operate the way nature intended.

Magnesium is also vital for proper heart function. It plays a recognized role in protecting against heart disease, including heart attacks, stroke, and hypertension (high blood pressure), which is clearly documented in hundreds of research studies. This fact is too often ignored by cardiologists, much to the detriment of their patients, and helps to explain why heart disease remains so prevalent worldwide, and in our society. A comprehensive meta-analysis, also published in 2012, brought this point home. The analysis examined previous studies involving more than 241,000 participants and found a "statistically significant inverse association between magnesium intake and risk of stroke." In other words, the less magnesium in your body, the greater your risk for stroke. (Larsson S, et al. 2012, Dietary

Magnesium intake and risk of stroke: a meta-analysis of prospective studies. *Am J Clin Nutr* 95(2): 269-270.)

Additional research has also shown that patients with low magnesium levels have a higher risk of dying of heart disease compared to patients with higher magnesium levels. Research shows that it acts as a natural calcium channel blocker, but without any of the health risks posed by calcium channel blocker drugs (Rosanoff A, Seelig MS. Comparison of mechanism and functional effects of Magnesium and statin pharmaceuticals. *J Am Coll Nutr.* 2004 Oct;23(5):501S-505S. PMID: 15466951), and also helps to prevent the formation of dangerous blood clots (Sheu JR, Hsiao G, et al. Antithrombotic effects of Magnesium sulfate in in vivo experiments. *Int J Hematol.* 2003 May;77(4):414-9. PMID: 12774935). Adequate levels of magnesium also help to regulate blood pressure levels and prevent high blood pressure (Guerrero-Romero F, Rodríguez-Morán M. Oral Magnesium supplementation with MgCl significantly reduces blood pressure in diabetic hypertensive adults with hypomagnesaemia. *J Hum Hypertens.* 2009 Apr;23(4):245-51. Epub 2008 Nov 20. PMID: 19020533), and protect against spasms in the arteries. And, of course, its role in Mg-ATP production is also essential for protecting the heart, since heart muscle cells contain very high concentrations of mitochondria that depend on ATP to do their non-stop functions.

Important as magnesium is for optimal heart function, however, it is copper that ensures that there is enough magnesium necessary for maintaining cardiovascular health and for carrying out its many other metabolic functions. This fact was established by the pioneering and penetrating research of Jerome L. Sullivan, MD, PhD (1944 to 2013), who introduced the concept of the "Iron-Heart Hypothesis" in a key research paper he published in the medical journal *Lancet* in 1981. (Sullivan JL, 1981, Iron and the sex difference in heart disease risk. *Lancet* 1:1293–4.) It is not hyperbole to say that Sullivan's research put the field of conventional cardiology on its ear. Every aspect of magnesium loss is caused by copper-iron dysregulation in the endothelial layer of the arteries and/or heart muscle cells (cardiomyocytes). This dysregulation causes increased oxidative stress, which then causes magnesium loss in the cells of those tissues. This is a particularly important concept to understand. Heart disease is not caused by a magnesium deficiency, per se. Rather, it is a fact that these cardiac issues are the result of copper deficiency causing an iron overload in the tissues of the heart and blood vessels. Yet, conventional cardiologists continue to debate Sullivan's findings while ignoring the mineral foundation of physiology.

In concluding this overview of magnesium, it is important to understand that, of all the minerals in the body, it is the one that is most rapidly depleted during times of stress. How quickly magnesium is depleted is best known as the "magnesium burn rate," or MBR. The key point to remember about MBR is that all of the negative stressors we experience in our day to day lives becomes oxidative stress inside our cells, and oxidative stress then eats magnesium for lunch. *(Please take a moment to re-read and reflect on that sentence some more.)* It is for this reason that daily and repeated supplementation of magnesium is such an integral part of the Root Cause Protocol. How to most effectively supplement with magnesium is explained in Chapter 9.

Ceruloplasmin: In the same way that the Sun is the center of our universe, I've come to regard ceruloplasmin as the 'Sun' of our bodily universe of metabolic activity. This most vital protein that expresses up to 20 or more enzyme functions that is produced in our livers, eyes, brains, kidneys, gonads, uterus, placenta, to name but a few of the key sites of synthesis.

To understand why ceruloplasmin is so important to our health, we need to consider how our body's cellular processes are designed to both produce energy and also to repair itself, contain, and eliminate toxins– including the toxic oxidants that are byproducts of energy production. As I previously pointed out, our cells need to be able to both create energy and clear "exhaust" as energy is produced by our mitochondrial power grid. This is one of the key roles that ceruloplasmin plays.

As the process of cellular respiration discussed above moves through its initial anaerobic first stage into its latter two aerobic stages to produce Mg-ATP, ceruloplasmin, along with other copper-dependent antioxidant enzymes keep in check the oxidants that are given off as byproducts of this process, preventing the oxidative stress that is the root cause of chronic conditions. Without ceruloplasmin, and the network of cupro-enzymes, the oxidants turn into free radicals that "rust" out tissues and organs. Keep in mind, the bulk of all of this activity takes place within our 40 quadrillion mitochondria.

Just as importantly, it is ceruloplasmin that makes copper available to our cells, tissues, and organs. An apt analogy is that ceruloplasmin is the "taxi" that drives copper to where copper needs to go. There is no greater need for copper than in our mitochondria (Frieden, 1985; Baker et al, 2017; Cobine et al, 2021).

This is hardly surprising since ceruloplasmin itself belongs to a family of protein/enzymes known as multicopper oxidases (MCOs). In this capacity, ceruloplasmin regulates the transportation of iron into red blood cells and other essential iron-containing proteins involved in cell growth. And, because ceruloplasmin is a carrier ("taxi") of copper—there are approximately six to eight atoms, or ions, of copper in each molecule of ceruloplasmin— ceruloplasmin, in combination with copper, controls iron metabolism and initiates the cell signaling pathways that help preventive oxidative stress and inflammation that iron would otherwise cause when it becomes unbound and unchecked in our cells and tissues. And it provides similar protection against unchecked oxygen. (Remember, oxygen acts as a double-edged sword to our cells. On the one hand, it is essential for the cells' energy and survival. On the other, if not properly regulated by ceruloplasmin and other key copper enzymes, oxygen can cause highly damaging free radicals.)

Ceruloplasmin's ability to both facilitate cellular energy production and prevent the formation of free radical oxidants is due to its shape and structure and the copper ions it contains that are involved in the giving and taking of electrons from oxygen, iron, and iron-binding proteins. Studies show that ceruloplasmin scavenge and inhibit the production of hydroxyl radicals, superoxide radicals, and lipid peroxides, all of which are types of oxidants that are dependent on iron ions. While we won't have the opportunity to expound further on these concepts in this book, it is worth noting that ceruloplasmin is pivotal for regulating iron, copper and oxygen status in the body. If energy is **falling** and oxidative stress is **rising**, then our body lacks bioavailable copper, or ceruloplasmin, as it is technically known. Tragically, the primal and pivotal roles for copper are simply not taught in any doctor school. As President Carter so aptly noted, *"Life is unfair."* This book, based upon my dedicated reading of hundreds of articles on copper metabolism, is my way of making life a bit more fair.

It is actually copper that is the key to the many ways that ceruloplasmin is able to maximize iron metabolism, acting through what is called ferroxidase, an enzyme that catalyzes iron to make sure that iron is not reactive. This fact is proven by research that shows defects or unhealthy mutations in the ceruloplasmin gene prevent copper from being naturally incorporated into ceruloplasmin, thereby disrupting iron metabolism and leading to iron accumulation. Studies have shown that defective ceruloplasmin, lacking copper, is a factor in a wide range of disease conditions. This can manifest as problems walking (gait abnormalities), impaired memory, speech problems, and other significant symptoms. (Sources for the above: Harris ZL, 2019, "Ceruloplasmin." Chapter 9 in *Clinical and Translation Perspective in Wilson Disease*. Academic Press; Pp 77-82; Poujois A, Poupon J and

Woimant F, 2019, "Direct Determination of Non-Ceruloplasmin-Bound Copper in Plasma" Chapter 22 in *Clinical and Translational Perspectives on Wilson Disease*. Academic Press; Pp249-255; Mateescu MA et al, 1998, Direct evidence of ceruloplasmin antioxidant properties. *Molecular and Cellular Biochemistry*. December DOI: 10.1023/A:1006945713860).

It is well chronicled in the medical literature that ceruloplasmin is the biological agent that is necessary to keep iron in a proper valence (meaning having the proper number of electrons in the outer shell), and, mostly importantly, to keep iron recycling around the body and the cell via key transport proteins. Scientists like to refer to this action as "cellular iron efflux," which is a fancy way of saying *"keep iron moving!"*

Circulating iron is the ideal state for iron. It is not meant to be stored. That is why measuring iron in its storage state, via the serum ferritin protein, makes little sense at all. It is akin to selecting a car based solely on the size of its trunk, while ignoring the size and efficiency of its engine. Who among us selects a car based on its trunk size? *No one!*

It is also known is that ceruloplasmin levels become elevated as an acute phase reactant in response to inflammation. This is a biological certainty that has been encoded into our bodies going back to the first appearance of humans on this planet. Yet, rather than recognizing that elevated ceruloplasmin, and the antioxidant actions of the copper ions that it carries, is an appropriate response by the body to infection/inflammation, Big Pharma is seeking to apply the same misinformation strategy to ceruloplasmin that it's done with cholesterol since 1955. Like cholesterol, they want us to see ceruloplasmin as the "bad guy," and recommend that we do what we can to "lower" it.

This makes absolutely no sense, because its elevation during an inflammatory state is a sign that ceruloplasmin is doing what it is meant to do, working to bring inflammation down and under control. Entirely missing in this drama is knowing the activity of this key protein. Knowing the level of ceruloplasmin is NOT the same as knowing its enzyme activity. There is a notable difference in measuring the height and the I.Q. of our children. Knowing the I.Q. of copper enzymes is a complete mystery in conventional and functional medicine. Doctors know the size of the "engine," but nothing about how fast, nor how far these "enzymes" can go. It is a glaring, but correctible blind spot.

What Pharma and physicians who accept this myth-guided approach are overlooking is that ceruloplasmin must have optimal levels of copper and that the amino acids be folded properly to function fully as the master antioxidant enzyme. As you might guess, the enzyme of choice is ferroxidase, which is one of the active components of ceruloplasmin that regulates iron status and iron movement in our body. Lowering ceruloplasmin totally disrupts this iron regulating process, leading to serious negative health consequences. As one scientific paper put it, *"It should be remembered that the protein (ceruloplasmin) is an acute phase entity so that its concentration in the plasma increases **twofold** to **threefold** [emphasis added[at the onset of infection or wounding. Under these circumstances, the multi-functionality may be highly important."* (Bento I. et al, 2007-Feb01, Ceruloplasmin revisited: structural and functional roles of various metal cation-binding sites. *Acta Crystallography D. Biol Crystallography; 63(Pt2): 240-248*). Based on everything I am learning about ceruloplasmin, I am confident in saying there is no "may" about it; ***ceruloplasmin's multi-functionality is highly important!***

Another example of ceruloplasmin's multi-functionality is the role it plays in helping the body fight infections. Like copper, ceruloplasmin is important for enabling neutrophils to kill harmful bacteria. In order for neutrophils to do so, iron has to be in a certain valence to turn off the activity of a key enzyme called myeloperoxidase (MPO) that can interfere with the ability of neutrophils to fight infection. Research proves that ceruloplasmin, by regulating iron valence, inhibits MPO. (Chapman ALP et al, 2013-Jan, Ceruloplasmin Is an Endogenous Inhibitor of Myeloperoxidase. *J Biol Chemistry*; 288: 6465-6477.) This is important because MPO promotes oxidative stress during inflammation and infection by producing a substance called hypochlorous acid (HOCl-). Ceruloplasmin acts as a protective shield against oxidant production by MPO because of its ability to regulate, or modulate the MPO response. It does this by managing iron so that it remains in the right state and stays active.

Ceruloplasmin's ability to keep MPO in check is also of significance to anyone who engages in endurance exercises, such as marathons. Endurance exercise depletes our minerals, especially magnesium. This depletion, in turn, sets the stage for an inflammatory response, including in the heart, and triggers a rise of MPO. In athletes who are short on ceruloplasmin, the degradation of heme that occurs as MPO becomes elevated releases more iron, which accelerates lipid peroxidation and overall oxidative stress, that invariably lowers magnesium status. In some cases, this can prove to be fatal for long distance runners, which explains why some of them die of heart attacks while running marathons, but always at the end of the race. (Melanson SEF et al, 2006-Dec, Elevation of Myeloperoxidase in Conjunction With Cardiac-Specific Markers After Marathon Running. *Amer J Clin Pathology*; 126(6): 888-893.)

Based on all of the above, you have a better understanding as to how and why copper, magnesium, and ceruloplasmin are so crucial for your health. To the extent that you feel the need, you might want to buy an extra copy of this book to broaden their scripted understanding of human physiology. Now let's revisit the process of cellular respiration so that we can understand how vitally important all three of these critical components are for optimal energy production.

Cellular Respiration Revisited

The quote by Douglas Wallace that opens this chapter is especially apt with regard to the cellular respiration process and the mitochondria. When you study the mitochondria, you soon come to realize how true Dr. Wallace's observation is. Everything to do with energy production by the mitochondria is indeed all about structure of these organelles and the flow of electrons through their respiratory complexes.

As I continually point out, in order to be healthy and energetic, our cells need to be able to both create energy *and* to clear exhaust, the resultant waste byproducts of making Mg-ATP. The challenge is that 90 percent of the energy, and 90 percent of the exhaust being produced is coming from our mitochondria. If the mitochondria are not properly structured, and if electrons are not properly flowing through them, then they're not going to activate oxygen cleanly and completely, and then we're going to get more exhaust building up, which will leave us more "exhausted" and, eventually, more chronically diseased. Preventing this "exhaustion" is the whole premise of the Root Cause Protocol, in a nutshell.

In the center of mitochondria is what is known as the matrix, which in appearance resembles a type of sea-colored swimming pool, and contains approximately 50,000 atoms of copper (Cobine et al, 2004; 2006). Why is that important? Because the mitochondria are the terminal destination points for both oxygen and iron, and it is copper that at the end of the day enables the mitochondria to create energy from oxygen and iron cleanly, while also effectively clearing the exhaust both oxygen and iron throw off as energy is produced. Copper is also instrumental in several of the respiratory complexes of the ETC (electron transport chain), and also for supporting the movement of ATP out of the mitochondria after it is produced. A lack of bioavailable copper impairs all of these processes. When we lose functional bioavailability of copper, we're left with a serious and cascading set of problems.

Now let's return to the actual process of how ATP is made. This occurs inside what is known as Complex IV of the mitochondria. Within Complex IV there is the movement of four electrons and four hydrogen protons. Oxygen is also coming in (although scientists do not know the exact mechanism; Wittenberg and Wittenberg, 2007), and water is going to be created and then ADP is going to be released. We start with O2 and then end with 2(H2O) as the activation process takes place in this key complex. The first step of that activation is that the di-oxygen molecule (O2) gets split. The second step is that the four electrons move through the complex. In the third step, the four hydrogens get pumped into the intermembrane space. And then, after the release of water, three ADP molecules get released and are transported over to Complex V, and this is where ADP becomes Mg-ATP.

All of this activity occurs by way of the unique electro-chemical properties of copper unique to MCOs (multi-copper oxidases). It's an evolutionary-conserved process that began billions of years ago. Electrons flow down through the membrane adjacent to the major copper pool in the mitochondrial matrix. When these actions do not happen completely or naturally with copper, we get "accidents with oxygen" that are called oxidants. Complex IV and Complex V are both copper-dependent. But what the research bears out is that when there's no copper available for the mitochondria, the entire mitochondria shut down, not just Complex IV and Complex V. If the mitochondria is lacking copper, they simply cannot function. This is not theory. There is extensive research to substantiate that statement.

Before discussing Complex IV further, I want to point out a very important fact about Complex I, one that was a game changer for me when I first became aware of it. Complex I is also known as NADH dehydrogenase, and NADH dehydrogenase is noted in a recent study as the second most prevalent copper protein/enzyme (also known as a cupro-protein) in the human body. This is NOT widely known and is significant because of NADH dehydrogenase's special importance to the first part of the overall ETC (electron transport chain). Specifically, it converts nicotinamide adenine dinucleotide (NAD) from its reduced form (NADH) to its oxidized form (NAD$^+$) to begin the process of ATP production.

In addition to catalyzing the transfer of electrons from NADH, it is essential for the normal functioning of all of the body's cells, including triggering apoptosis (natural programmed cell death), thus helping to prevent cancer. Moreover, defects and mutations in NADH dehydrogenase have been linked to a wide range of inherited neuromuscular and metabolic conditions, as well as heart attack and stroke. (Chomova M, Racay P, 2010-Mar, Mitochondrial complex I in the network of known and unknown facts. *General Physiology and Biophysics; 29 (1): 3–11).*

Complex I and the other four cytochrome protein complexes are composed of heme proteins, which means that they contain ferrous (Fe2+) iron, the most reactive form of iron. This critical cytochrome c oxidase enzyme does not work without bioavailable copper, which is the key to making these ATP-producing engines work. What do you think is supplying the copper energy for this critical aspect of our metabolism? Ceruloplasmin! (Broderius M, et al, 2010-May, Levels of plasma ceruloplasmin protein are markedly lower following dietary copper deficiency in rodents. *Comp Biochem Physiol Pharmacol C Toxicol Pharmacol; 151(4):473-479)* www.ncbi.nlm.nih.gov/pmc/articles/PMC2854028/pdf/nihms-192848.pdf)

Also note that oxidative stress is being given off on both sides of the mitochondrial process of energy production. Oxidative stress is a natural byproduct of these activities, but as copper levels drop, due to increased stressors, there is an obligate increase in the oxidative stress. It is axiomatic. It is biologic. The greatest source of cellular oxidative stress occurs across these critical energy-producing actions of the respiratory complexes I through to V, especially when copper is marginal in the diet and deficient in the tissue. When was the last time your doctor discussed, much less measured, your copper status?

It is common to think that only copper/zinc superoxide dismutase (Cu/Zn-SOD), also known as SOD I, work the intracellular space (i.e. outside the mitochondria), and that only manganese superoxide dismutase (Mn-SOD), also known as SOD II, only works the intra-mitochondrial membrane (i.e. inside the mitochondria). I used to think that was the case, too, until I learned more about ceruloplasmin by reading a study entitled "Ceruloplasmin: A Scavenger of Superoxide Anion Radicals". (Goldstein IM et al, 1979-May, *The Journal of Biological Chemistry*; 254(10): 4040-4045.) That's when I learned that the ceruloplasmin's ferroxidase enzyme is a recognized scavenger of superoxide radicals, reactive oxygen molecules that are quite destructive, and which can and do devolve both inside and outside the mitochondria. They can also turn into the most destructive molecule on the planet, the hydroxyl radical ($\cdot$OH). This is the metabolic origin of what dings DNA (deoxyribonucleic acid) to create epigenetic chaos to bring about MTHFR (methylenetetrahydrofolate reductase) and other notable gene defects. This destructive molecule also leads to a breakdown in the efficiency and impact of the energy production of mitochondria, causing chronic fatigue syndrome (CFS), as well a host of other chronic conditions of low energy, and disrupting the cellular machinery of key aspects of our physiology, like the liver, heart, brain, kidneys, joints, muscles, and adipocytes.

Furthermore, ceruloplasmin is not just restricted to the cytoplasm (i.e. outside the mitochondria). This superoxide radical scavenger is also found inside the mitochondria, as well. (Vasin AV et al, 2005. Mitochondrial ceruloplasmin of mammals. *Molecular Biology* 39:42-45 www.ncbi.nlm.nih.gov/m/pubmed/15773547; Balevska P et al, 1975, Studies on the transfer of copper from ceruloplasmin to mitochondria. *Agressologie*, 16 Spec No. C:7-11 www.ncbi.nlm. nih.gov/m/pubmed/1232838/) This fact, coupled with the fact we learned above, ceruloplasmin is the "taxi" that transports copper to where it is needed inside the mitochondria, is more proof of how essential adequate supplies of both copper and ceruloplasmin are for healthy energy production. I guarantee, you will be hard pressed to find a doctor today who pays attention to, or was properly trained in these foundational cupro-facts. If you want more energy and less exhaustion, I'm quite confident that more bioavailable copper is your ticket to both!

And the roles above are not the only one's copper and ceruloplasmin play in energy production. It turns out that 20 percent of the mitochondrial bi-lipid membrane is made up of a phospholipid called cardiolipin, which is a fat that enables proper electron transport chain function. While cardiolipin is 20 percent of the total composition of mitochondria, it is actually 50 percent of the phospholipids found to be a part of the ETC lipids (i.e. respiratory complexes I – IV). (Soussi B, et al,1990-Jan, "1H-n.m.r. evaluation of the ferricytochrome c-cardiolipin interaction: Effect of superoxide radicals" *Biochem Jrl* 265(1):227-232. www.ncbi.nlm.nih.gov/pmc/ articles/PMC1136634/pdf/biochemj00192-0227.pdf)

Cardiolipin is essential for the function of cytochrome c oxidase (Complex IV). Copper is the key to start this cytochrome c oxidase enzyme production of ATP. Cardiolipin is the fuel upon which the cytochrome c oxidase enzyme works. And, as one scientific study points out about the origin of mitochondrial dysfunction: *"Mitochondrial dysfunction… is related to a decreased cytochrome c oxidase activity, ultimately because of cardiolipin peroxidation [i.e. rusting of the fats] causing a diminished cytochrome c binding to this enzyme."* (Smith et al, 1980; Okayasu et al, 1985) And that's what leads to the breakdown of both mitochondrial function and the ability of minerals, especially copper and magnesium, to create the cellular and mitochondrial matrix substrates, that are required for the natural and sustainable creation of ATP.

In the absence, or the presence of lowered production, of ceruloplasmin, those ubiquitous superoxide ($*O2-$) molecules get furthered radicalized by ferrous ($Fe2+$) iron and turn into the OH-radical that then oxidizes the cardiolipin. I happen to think it is relevant and most vital that ceruloplasmin brings both the copper (key) and ensures that the cardiolipin (fuel) does not get "rusty," as we explored the car analogy earlier in this chapter. Ceruloplasmin, as the ferroxidase enzyme, converts ferrous ($Fe2+$) iron into ferric ($3+$) iron. It is this latter form of iron that can then be used in cellular transport and other metabolic proteins to keep us healthy and energized. Isn't it amazing that one protein, ceruloplasmin, does all of this? Yet, you've never heard its name.

But, as they say, "there's more." Another important and interesting fact about human biology and biochemistry is that T3, the active thyroid hormone, acts as an oxygen sensor in the body, helping to ensure that oxygen is being burned ("activated") cleanly, therefore not causing excess oxidation. If this is not the case, this critical hormone sends a message signaling the liver to make more ceruloplasmin (Mittag J et al, 2012-Apr, Serum Copper as a Novel Biomarker for resistance to Thyroid Hormone. *Biochem Jrl* 443(1):103-109).

To sum up, we lose the ability to transport copper because we don't have access to the ceruloplasmin taxi, which feeds copper to the cells and to the mitochondria. If ceruloplasmin cannot get copper to the cells and their mitochondrial power grids, the result is a general breakdown of ATP production. And if enough copper is not available, we cannot regulate oxygen metabolism and cytochrome c oxidase is not going to be able to activate oxygen to create energy. If that happens, then we're not going to be able to regulate iron metabolism. The end result is that our mitochondria are not able to make energy, and the body is not going to be able to make heme and iron sulfur clusters, which are created as a part of the mitochondrial actions. Given that iron is a terminal destination in the mitochondria, we're going to have a serious problem because this iron will build up inside the ferritin storage proteins, both inside the mitochondria, as well as inside the cells. Then we're going to lose the ability to regulate the reactive oxidative stress that takes place. And we're not going to have enough antioxidant enzymes to break down the oxidative stress that's building. This is why both copper and ceruloplasmin are so important for proper energy production that does not result in iron buildup and oxidative stress, particularly in Complex IV, but in all mitochondrial complexes of the ETC.

Now let's take a look at the roles magnesium plays in this overall process. Inside our body, energy is spelled Mg-ATP. The body can't recognize ATP, and the body cannot use it unless that magnesium molecule is properly attached. That's why magnesium is also found within the mitochondrial matrix, alongside of copper.

Magnesium is also vital for maintaining proper calcium homeostasis. Without adequate magnesium levels, calcium levels become unregulated and unbalanced. Many within the field of modern medicine would have you believe that calcium is running the show, and not magnesium. That is absolutely not the case. However, calcium can have a very decided controlling, negative impact on mitochondria if its levels get too high inside of cells. That said, what causes the unchecked release of calcium into the cell? Rising oxidative stress from iron accumulation!

Within the process of glycolysis that occurs during the prep stage of cellular respiration, glycogen that becomes glucose is being chopped up. Think of scissors. Glycolysis is chopping up glucose into 3-carbon component parts called pyruvate. As we've discussed, the process of glycolysis is anaerobic, meaning it takes place without oxygen and occurs within the cytosol, outside of the mitochondria. What's particularly important about this is that the pyruvate are turned into the high energy electron carriers NADH, and FADH2 along with hydrogen atoms. It is these hydrogen atoms that "run the pump" at Complex V so that ATP is produced.

As we have discussed, both hydrogen *and* oxygen need to be activated so that hydrogen is oxidized and electrons are taken away from it. At the same time, oxygen is being reduced as the electrons taken from hydrogen are added to it. These chemical changes are what makes water, and they are essential to create ATP. The late, great Guy E. Abraham, MD, was able to demonstrate the importance of magnesium to all of these different components of the anaerobic process of turning glycogen into pyruvate. This is a big deal. Magnesium is very important to this process. Magnesium isn't involved in all of the steps, but most of the steps by far are dependent on magnesium to activate the enzymes that turn glucose or glycogen into pyruvate.

Then, as cellular respiration continues in the Krebs cycle, many enzymes are involved, but the critical enzymes are also dependent on magnesium. These enzymes are known as dehydrogenase enzymes, and are so named because they take hydrogen away from substances. The way to think of this is that magnesium is what enables the substrates—the building parts, if you will—to carry out their roles in producing ATP. The substrates are solely dependent on magnesium to be able to be available for use by the electron transport chain.

Once pyruvate is produced in the cytosol, it needs to move into the mitochondria, where it can become acetyl-CoA via an enzyme known as pyruvate dehydrogenase. If there is a buildup of oxidative stress in the cell, pyruvate cannot become acetyl-CoA. If magnesium is not available because there is too much oxidative stress, the pyruvate will become lactic acid, a process triggered by the enzyme lactate dehydrogenase. If that happens, you're going to be left with a very low energy production. The reason why Dr. Abraham was so obsessed with this was because he was trying to crack the code of fibromyalgia, which is characterized by low energy. One of his signature discoveries was how important magnesium is to the process of making pyruvate and then getting it into the mitochondria. The mitochondrial pyruvate channel is entirely magnesium dependent. (Abraham GE et al, 1992, "Management of Fibromyalgia: Rationale for the Use of Magnesium and Malic Acid" *Jrl Nutr Med* 3:49-59.)

Magnesium is also important for the activity of isocitrate dehydrogenase (IDH), which is considered the rate limiting enzyme of the Krebs or citric acid cycle. IDH catalyzes an oxidation reduction that turns isocitrate, a substrate of the citric acid cycle, into oxalosuccinate, helping to make NADH from NAD, and making hydrogen protons available. If that doesn't happen, then we have a real breakdown in energy production in the cell.

Again, there are three stages to making ATP—glycolysis, the TCA/Krebs cycle, and then the ETC (electron transport chain). Copper, ceruloplasmin and magnesium are all essential for all three stages. Yet most doctors are unaware of and have not been trained in any of these three, leaving their chronically fatigued patients to wander the halls of the Internet looking for answers and never having the energy they need to become and to stay healthy.

Mitochondrial Dysfunction is *Not* The Cause of Low Energy

Earlier in this chapter, I mentioned Denham Harman, PhD, MD, whose free radical theory of aging gave us the understanding we have today about how accidents with oxygen (oxidants aka free radicals) can and do impair our health and accelerate the aging process. However, after spending years trying and failing to increase maximum human lifespan, Harman became frustrated and dug deeper. After additional research, he concluded that mitochondria are not only damaged by oxidative stress, but produce free radicals, as well, just as I've explained above. He also concluded that it is the health and functioning of mitochondria that determine our lifespan. He published his theory, known today as the "mitochondrial theory of aging" in the April 1972 issue of the *Journal of the American Geriatrics Society*. (Harman, D, 1972, "A biologic clock: the mitochondria?" *J American Geriatrics Society;* 20 (4): 145–147).

For years, Harman's additional research was overlooked by modern medicine, but in recent years more and more practitioners and scientists are now talking about "mitochondrial dysfunction." Among the phrases that chafe me, I regard "mitochondrial dysfunction" to be among the most offensive. To me, it is a term that conjures up an equal amount of fear and confusion, much like that often-used phrase, *"You have a lesion."* (What *exactly* is that?!?)

There are thousands of articles, both for the layperson and for the doctor and scientist, written about this mitochondrial condition that is rapidly becoming a pandemic on this planet. Yet, when all the dust settles, they are akin to articles about how to drive a car, providing meticulous detail to every facet of that automotive experience with the notable exclusion of two key and fundamental dimensions for a successful car ride:

- *Forgetting to tell you that it's really important to bring a key to start the engine*
- *Forgetting to tell you that the engine must have fuel to keep it running*

Even though this term, "mitochondrial dysfunction," seems hopeless, and although it *is* a critical issue we all recognize and know, it *is not* the real heart of the problem. When whittled down to size and made far easier to comprehend and understand, then we can prevent or reverse its development in our metabolism, which is exactly what the Root Cause Protocol is designed to do.

Doctors fail to do this for the simple reason that they do not know how.

Why?

Because they have not been trained to look in the right places.

A basic mantra in business school is, *"What gets measured, gets managed."* The first rule of management is that you can't improve that which is not observed, nor measured. What physicians fail to observe, let alone measure and therefore manage, is the status of their patients' copper, magnesium, and ceruloplasmin levels. Again, they have not been trained to look at these factors. Moreover, there is a total absence of medical training about how to measure mitochondrial activity, or how to make mitochondria more vital.

As I shared earlier, we have 40 quadrillion mitochondria in our body, distributed across many diverse cell types. Physicians rarely consider this fact, if they are even aware of it to begin with. And they often overlook the importance of cardiolipin, which, as I explained, is a fat that enables proper electron transport chain function. When there's a buildup of oxidative stress in the cell, cardiolipin gets peroxidized ("rusty"). Oxidative stress is what leads to the breakdown of mitochondrial function, impairing the ability of essential minerals, especially copper and magnesium, to create cellular and matrix substrates, and then enable the creation of ATP.

And then there is the fact that there are ten times more defects in mitochondrial DNA than in nuclear DNA. Very few doctors talk about that. Nor do they talk about the fact that 90 percent of the oxidative stress in our bodies is taking place inside the mitochondria. Again, we're back to structure and energy. If the structure of the mitochondria begins to falter because of the change in the genetic expression of mitochondrial DNA due to a loss of energy caused oxidative stress, then everything else in the body is negatively impacted.

The root cause of all of this is our lifelong battle with oxygen, keeping it in check so that our cells, tissues, and organs have all of the oxygen they need, but no more, so that they do not begin to rust out. It is our bioavailable copper regulating these dynamics in ALL of our cells. This is a very important concept to understand and to internalize.

It is tied in with mitochondrial function and the fact that as we age the level of iron and the levels of copper and magnesium begin to crisscross. Iron is building up from cradle to grave and copper is doing just the opposite. There is ample research that backs these dynamics up. Magnesium is falling as well, but in terms of the real payoff for energy production in our mitochondria, it is bioavailable copper that we are most dependent upon.

That is why the term "mitochondrial dysfunction" chafes me. Despite what doctors may claim, mitochondrial dysfunction is NOT a disease. Rather, and most importantly, it is a classic clinical sign of mineral dysregulation, which is the *real* root cause problem, pure and simple. Specifically, a dysregulation, or lack of, bioavailable copper, magnesium, and ceruloplasmin—the three most essential and more valuable workhorses necessary for mitochondrial health and function, as well as optimal energy. Solving this mineral dysregulation is not only the most effective way to ensure that we have all of the energy our body needs, it is in fact *the only natural and sustainable way*!

Now that we understand how our body really produces energy, let's examine why the concentration on iron by doctors for their patients' lack of energy is so misguided. That is the focus of Chapter 4.

Oxidation: The Medical Profession's Iron-ic Blind Spot

"...but the simplest thing cannot be made clear to the most intelligent man if he is firmly persuaded that he knows already, without a shadow of a doubt, what is laid before him."

– Leo Tolstoy

"It's not what you don't know that's the problem. It's what you know, for certain, that just ain't so."

– Mark Twain

"What we already know is a great hindrance into discovering the unknown."

– Claude Bernard, MD (1813–1878)

"None can destroy Iron, but its own rust can. Likewise, none can destroy a person, but his own mindset can."

– Ratan Tata

In the last chapter, we learned that copper makes energy and iron takes it. In this chapter, you will learn exactly how and why iron steals energy and why chronic fatigue and anemia are not due to an iron deficiency, despite what doctors and modern medicine have been telling us for so long. You will also learn why excess iron in the tissue, not in the blood, is the major culprit that causes oxidative stress and robs us of our mitochondrial energy production. Even though practitioners rarely mention this to their patients, iron overload is now known to be a central causative factor in a wide range of disease conditions (Weinberg E, 2010), including:

Abdominal Pain

Adrenal Function Problems

Alzheimer's disease, Dementia, Parkinson's, and other neurodegenerative diseases

Amenorrhea (Loss of Period)

Atherosclerosis, Arrhythmia, Heart Attack, and other cardiovascular diseases

Autoimmune Disorders

Blood Sugar Dysregulation (Hypoglycemia)

Cancer

Chronic Fatigue

Depression

Enlarged Spleen

Hair Loss

Hepatitis C

Hypogonadism

Hypopituitarism

Hypothyroidism

Impotence

Infertility

Low Libido/Loss of Interest in Sex

Non-alcoholic fatty liver disease, Cirrhosis of the liver, and other liver conditions

Osteoporosis and Osteopenia

Rheumatoid Arthritis, Osteoarthritis, and Joint Pain

Sarcopenia (muscle wasting)

Skin Color Changes (Bronze, Ashen-Gray, Green)

Type 2 Diabetes and Metabolic syndrome

While I'm well aware of these known connections with iron overload, most people and their practitioners are not, despite the published findings of acclaimed researchers such as E.D. Weinberg, PhD; Leo R. Zacharski, MD; George Bartzokis, MD; Douglas B. Kell, PhD; James F. Collins, PhD; and Robert R. Crichton, PhD, and many others. Their work informs much of what we will learn in this chapter.

To set the stage for this discussion, let me start by stating that while we know what we know, *we don't know what we don't know.* This is a very important premise for introducing new thought. We can moan about what practitioners don't know, but they simply don't know what they don't know. And we don't know what we don't know, either. So, though the information in this chapter—indeed, throughout this entire book—may be new to you, please come to it with an open mind. As for our doctors, we must understand that they were not trained to know these mineral and metabolic dynamics. Now, we might quibble with them regarding their limited curiosity to better understand why their patients are constantly stressed and fatigued, but we should not fault them for their narrow and scripted training.

Let me also state that, if people knew how little practitioners know about mineral metabolism, oxygen metabolism, and energy metabolism, they would probably never go to see their doctor. But because we and our doctors don't know about these three dynamics, we have been "trained" to believe in disease. And that's the basis of the whole dynamic that is fueling our national/global health crisis. Add to that the wisdom of my friend, Pastor Joey Foster, who teaches a course in logic. The cornerstone of this course is that *missing information equals missing truth*. When I first heard that phrase, there was a seismic shift in my understanding of these issues. This "missing information" is what has been ruling the world of medicine since its founding at the Royal College of Physicians and Surgeons in 1518. There is a great deal of missing information, and we're just now beginning to connect the mineral and metabolic dots to discover what's been left out or overlooked during these past 500 years.

Let's explore oxygen first, specifically the oxidative stress that occurs inside our body as oxygen is used to help produce energy and water inside the mitochondria during the process of cellular respiration that we learned about previously in Chapter 3.

Oxygen Is Good, "Oxy-Dents" Are Very Bad

Oxidative stress is a fancy way of saying "rust." I also think of this form of stress as an "accident with oxygen" or an "oxy-dent." Just as we do not want rust and dents to affect our car, so too do we not want our cells, tissues, and organs to "rust" or become "dented". Yet, it is a biological fact that, throughout our lives, we are in a perpetual battle with oxygen, as well as iron, with both oxidative stress and unbound iron increasing inside of our bodies as we age. Neil Young got it right: "*Rust never sleeps.*"

It is a biological fact that oxygen is the second most reactive element on the planet. Iron is considered the master pro-oxidant element on the planet. When they mix, whether outside or inside our body, "rust" and physical degeneration will follow. This is the basis of the "Free Radical Theory" conceived of and promoted by Denham Harman, PhD, MD in 1956, which we explored in Chapter 3.

Our existence on the planet is based on balancing energy and exhaust. And what is important to understand is that we are surrounded by poison in the air. It's called oxygen. Is the oxygen molecule the protagonist of our story, or is it the antagonist? That depends on which way you look at it. In Chapter 3 you learned that the processing of oxygen inside the mitochondria both creates 90 percent of the energy (protagonist), but it also creates 90 percent of the exhaust (antagonist). To stay healthy, we seek to keep both that energy production<>exhaust elimination in regular balance, and be able to clear that metabolic exhaust. Being able to use oxygen to metabolize our food is what allows us to be a higher order species, and is something that occurred through evolution. The magic of oxygen is that it takes the glucose and fat in food and facilitates a 20- to 70-fold increase in ATP production compared to anaerobic metabolism that was how energy was produced before oxygen appeared in the atmosphere several billion years ago.

As we get older, we have increased oxidative stress, or "rust," and that rusting process is taking place inside our body. We know that we can't live without oxygen, but equally true is that we also cannot age without oxidants ("oxy-dents"). Tied in with this is the daily and ongoing buildup of iron as we move through life. As babies, we start out with a little bit of iron, and then we add an average of one milligram of iron every day that we are alive. That iron mixes with oxygen to create oxidative stress. As a result, our cellular energy diminishes as we get older. The world-renowned iron biologists Crichton, Gutteridge and Halliwell, Kell, Collins, Weinberg and others all know and regularly write about this.

For most people, the midpoint of this process occurs around the age of 40. That's when everything starts to change in our energy level and health issues start to become chronic and more noticeable. One of the first indications of this, by the way, is that people in their 40s begin to experience changes in their eyesight. That's an early warning sign that oxidative stress is building, even if doctors don't pick up on it. Fatigue, as well as aches and pains usually set in around this time, too. Given the known connection between eye health and liver health documented within the annals of TCM (Traditional Chinese Medicine), this change in visual acuity should be an important clue to practitioners that their clients' iron status, and thus, their overall health status is indeed changing.

Sadly, many people today are developing chronic oxidative stress and higher iron buildup well before they turn 40, due to the environmental and dietary factors that we examined in Chapter 2. There have been some very profound changes made in our food system since World War II, many that we're not even fully aware of. We've never really connected all the dots. But we do know that commercial farming has had a very significant impact on the availability of minerals in the soil, and that since 1941 iron has been added to our food and, in the US, was further increased by 50 percent in 1969 (Moon, 2008), principally in the wheat and grain products that are so prevalent in the standard Western diet. And it is NOT organic iron that is being added to "fortify" or "enrich" our food; it is iron filings! (For those of you who are intrigued by this, you can see videos on YouTube where people have taken cereal, ground it up, put it in their milk, and then place a magnet in it to literally pull the iron-laden cereal out of the bowl. This is only possible because of the iron filings these cereals contain. That form of toxic iron is going inside our bodies, and it is immediately turned in to "rust." It's important that we be mindful of that fact. More importantly, we need to take action to curb this intake of "enriched" foods.)

As oxidative stress takes hold within our bodies, normal cells begin to devolve. During cellular respiration, oxygen becomes superoxide and then hydrogen peroxide that, under the right anti-oxidant conditions, becomes water. Notably, it is copper that enables those transactions to occur safely, while blocking the creation of the hydroxyl radical, which is the most destructive biomolecule on the planet. Without copper, we will have this oxidative injury and cell damage. In scientific terms, this is known as redox cycling pathology. It's just as accurate to think of it as rust.

Recapping what happens during the aerobic stages of cellular respiration, one molecule of oxygen (O_2) turns into two molecules of water ($2H_2O$) via the transfer of four electrons from NADH and four hydrogen protons ($H+$) to an O_2 molecule that occurs in the ETC (electron transport chain) of the mitochondria. These key reactions are catalyzed by the copper-rich enzyme, cytochrome c oxidase (aka, Complex IV). When optimal levels of copper are present in this Complex IV, there are minimal levels of oxidants (ROS) given off and the oxidants are metabolized and scavenged by the mitochondrial and cellular antioxidant enzymes that also run on the energy of copper (SOD, CAT, GPx, PON-1, etc.).

However, without enough bioavailable copper, oxygen molecules can interact with respiratory enzyme complexes earlier in the ETC (electron transport chain), and can create especially the reactive oxygen species superoxide ($*O_2-$) and hydrogen peroxide (H_2O_2), both of which can then react with and damage proteins and unsaturated fatty acids that are pervasive in the cells, tissues and organs of the body. An even more serious problem arises if the hydrogen peroxide finds a free iron ion. When that happens, hydrogen peroxide and iron combine to catalyze the production of hydroxyl radicals ($\cdot OH$), which are extremely reactive and very damaging, ensuring a loss of energy, causing lipid peroxidation, dinging mitochondrial and nuclear DNA, and creating changes in structure and function of proteins and amino acids. This is the very essence of "mitochondrial dysfunction" that we discussed previously.

It is a scientific fact that oxidation ("rust") causes structural changes inside the body. As soon as oxygen cannot be activated and turned into water to release ADP in the ETC (electron transport chain), it becomes ROS that oxidizes molecules around it by changing their structure. ***ATP and ROS are flip-sides of the same O2 coin!*** And as bioavailable copper becomes more deficient and dysfunctional, iron becomes more prevalent and more destructive.

Therein lies the acceleration of aging and chronic conditions. It is THAT basic.

It is the copper-rich enzymes within the mitochondria and the cells that prevent all of this from happening. They do so by quickly reducing and removing free radicals. In other words, by clearing the metabolic exhaust **before** it can cause rust in the surrounding tissue(s). It is bioavailable copper that keeps the energy and the exhaust in proper balance. We humans, as well as all other aerobic life on this planet, must have bioavailable copper in order to survive and thrive (Cobine P, 2017). That is not taught in doctor school, but that's the whole basis of the Root Cause Protocol and the RCP Institute that trains practitioners to think "energetically!"

The Crux of the Problem

I'm very focused on the ***why***.

I started my research many years ago with two key questions. The first question was, *Why is everyone so sick?* My stock and trade activity during the years I spent as a consultant for hospitals was forecasting disease indexes, and determining what the demand for healthcare services were going to be so that hospitals could most effectively grow to meet those demands.

I was pretty good at it.

The other question that emerged, as I learned more and more about anemia, was: *How could anemia exist when iron is the number one element on the planet?* As I mentioned, ~35 percent of the Earth's composition is comprised of iron, yet iron deficiency anemia is claimed to be the number one nutrient deficiency among humans (WHO, 2010). That didn't make sense to me. It didn't pass any sniff test at all. That would mean that the most evolved species on the planet had lost the natural ability to metabolize the #1 element on the planet. That made NO sense to me at all.

To find the answers to those questions, I disciplined myself to spend two to three hours every morning, seven days a week, scouring the medical literature, which is something I continue to do to this day, more than a decade later. I began to piece together the explanation for those whys, looking for points of intersection and synthesis. (If I have any analytical gift, it is pattern recognition.) What has become crystal clear is that the answers I was seeking to help people have more energy and eliminate their fatigue lay within the body's enzyme systems, especially those that run on the energy and "intellect" of copper! Despite the assertions otherwise, I'm confident that the body does not run on hormones. It runs on enzymes. (Case in point: EVERY hormone on this planet is made with enzymes!) There are about 9,000 enzymes in the body and they all work just like the cars we drive. Key question: When was the last time you drove your car without a key? Unless you're Fred or Wilma Flintstone, it's simply not possible.

As I've come to conclude, there is a hierarchy to the 92 known minerals on this planet, and there are two minerals that act as principal "keys" to many of these 9000 enzymes: bioavailable copper and magnesium. That's just staggering to think about.

But what's even more amazing is that both of these minerals are lost to stress, especially magnesium via acute stress and copper under conditions of chronic stress. Magnesium and B-vitamins are the nutrients that disappear the fastest in the human body in response to acute stress. I refer to this dynamic as the magnesium burn rate, or MBR. When you feel that knot in your stomach because you've got a deadline or you've got some major bill due or you've had an argument with your spouse or you are experiencing any other type of stress in your life, magnesium is leaving your body very quickly. And magnesium is connected to 3,751 enzymes in the human body. (Piovesan et al, 2012-Sep07, "The Human 'Magnesome': Detecting Magnesium Binding Sites on Human Proteins". *BMC Bioinformatics13* (Suppl 14): S10) We'll talk more about this dynamic in Chapter 6.

From solely a mineral perspective, in today's UBER-stressed world, we need more magnesium, we need more bioavailable copper, and we also need less iron in our diet. Ceruloplasmin is important too because when it disappears, you lose metabolic homeostasis, the ability to express these copper-dependent enzymes, and what is "myth diagnosed" as "anemia of iron deficiency" is, for a fact, "anemia of iron dysregulation" or as it is classified clinically, "anemia of chronic disease" or "anemia of inflammation." Missing ferroxidase enzyme expression by ceruloplasmin leads to many disease conditions as our body becomes starved for proper iron recycling, because it is really starved for bioavailable copper. When that happens, the concept of "anemia of chronic disease" emerges, and it has been proven to be from a copper deficiency that affects the iron recycling system in our bodies. (Cartwright and Wintrobe, 1952, "Anemia of Infection. XVII: A Review" *Adv Intern Med* 5: 165-226; DeDemonico et al, 2008; Musci et al, 2014.)

As you know from reading this far, increasing and maintaining bioavailable copper, magnesium, and ceruloplasmin, while keeping iron in check, are the priorities of the Root Cause Protocol, to ensure proper mineral focus for energy and exhaust management within our mitochondria. When you begin to think about the incredible complexity and sophistication of one mitochondrion and then consider the 40 quadrillion mitochondria that are found in our body's

100 trillion cells, it becomes obvious that we are in essence "mineral beings," but we've never known that. That truth has been buried in all of the terminology and articles that are used by laypersons and health professionals alike when discussing human physiology and health conditions. Minerals are regarded as a "hood ornament," at best, and NOT the "keys" that start the engines (enzymes).

The relentless and ever-occurring magnesium loss is caused by this iron accumulation because there is a torturous relationship between iron and magnesium in our cells, tissues and organs. Then, when we come back to the process of energy loss, we find again that too much iron is the culprit. When you introduce too much iron into the mitochondria, the medial literature wants you to believe that it's very tightly regulated. It simply is not, certainly NOT in the modern era of low bioavailable copper and high iron fortification. ATP production can vary by at least 40 percent and as much as 96 percent if there's too much iron in the cell and/or in the mitochondria. *This "stuck" iron is the metabolic stimulus for inflammation.*

Inflammation does not come from Mars and furthermore, it is NOT a disease. It comes from inside iron toxic cells because iron triggers interleukin 6 (IL-6), which triggers the release of hepcidin, which is considered the iron regulatory hormone. In fact, hepcidin is called the "hormone of inflammation." And when bioavailable copper, in the form of ferroxidase enzyme at the "iron doorway" (ferroportin) is missing, hepcidin will inevitably rise and so, too, will iron remain stuck inside the cell. Please know, I am merely providing some headlines to this intricate and delicate facet of iron metabolism. There is way more to this iron-y than can be presented in this book.

Despite these known scientific facts, when you read most articles about iron, you will find they state that iron is the #1 nutrient deficiency on planet Earth. The World Health Organization (WHO) insists this is the case, as well, and claims that as many as two billion people are now "iron deficient." ***Please do not confuse iron deficiency with iron dysregulation,*** an all too familiar mistake made in clinical circles. Furthermore, please do not confuse iron *in the blood* (i.e., a blood test) with iron *in the tissue*. Rarely is this assessment of the distinction ever done by any doctor. There is a major difference in iron's status in these two settings inside our body.

When I read statements like that, or that G6PD, which is a very important enzyme inside the red blood cell, is the #1 enzyme deficiency, my tendency, being curious by nature, is to say, "Let's dig a little deeper." And that's exactly what we're going to do.

It turns out that iron deficiency isn't the actual issue. The real problem is that, due to the dietary and environmental factors that have depleted our bodies of copper, magnesium, and ceruloplasmin over the past century, we modern humans are not able to metabolize, or process, iron the way MTHR Nature intended. In scientific terms, this means that our bodies are becoming increasingly unable to maintain proper iron homeostasis. As a result, we experience chronic unbound iron that reacts badly with oxygen (Kell DB, 2009a), saddling us with the ravages of oxidative stress. This quote from a 2001 research paper published in the *Brain Research Bulletin* sums things up perfectly: *"The underlying pathogenic event in oxidative stress is cellular iron mismanagement."* (Thompson KI et al, 2001-May, "Iron & Neurologic Disorders." **Brain Res Bull** 55(2):155-64.)

As we've noted, there are two states of valence for iron: $Fe(2+)$, called ferrous iron, and $Fe(3+)$, called ferric iron. Because there was no oxygen in Earth's atmospheric and ancient past, iron, because of its dominance on the planet, was very important for sustaining life, which at that time was completely anaerobic. Iron has four unpaired electrons in its structure, and also has the capacity to share electrons, which is very significant. When oxygen finally began to appear some 3.4 billion years ago, the biochemical dynamics of iron changed because of how iron reacts with oxygen.

What I find fascinating is that there really isn't iron metabolism or copper metabolism, per se. ***There is only copper-iron metabolism and both metals are joined at the hip by ceruloplasmin,*** the key copper protein that regulates the valence of both iron and copper, and provides a spectrum of antioxidant enzymes to our bodies as our need arises. Together, iron and copper act as a kind of ventriloquist act in which iron is the dummy, and copper is the one calling the metabolic shots in our body, contrary to what you may think or your practitioner has been "trained" to think. I have learned to think of iron as "*inert*," and copper as "*intelligent*."

As we've noted previously, iron in our body is used to carry oxygen via hemoglobin. If we don't have the hemoglobin moving the oxygen to where it needs to go, we are in trouble. But it turns out that in the human body, for every atom of copper, there are 60 atoms of iron. Again, it is copper that is calling the shots, just as it is that the chef, not the waiters, is most important asset to the success of any fine restaurant. There is only one mineral that carries oxygen. That's iron. But there's only one mineral that activates and harnesses oxygen, and that's copper!

Here is another very important point to remember:

Dysregulated, unbound, excess iron is the greatest source of oxidative stress and inflammation in the body. This fact is well understood by iron biologists, not so much by clinicians treating the symptoms of tissue iron overload.

Which is not to say that iron is not important to our health. It is vitally important. It is when it becomes unbound and ends up where it does not belong in the body that problems arise in our physiology. And the problems go far beyond fatigue, as the list of chronic conditions associated with iron overload highlighted at the beginning of this chapter makes abundantly clear.

Iron's Roles in the Body as Intended by Nature

Iron is not only found in hemoglobin, it is needed to produce it. In addition, because of its ability to transport oxygen, iron is playing a role in helping to maintain immune function, ensure that muscles function and contract properly, improve endurance, maintains lung health and proper respiration, and repairs damaged cells, tissues and organs. Iron is also a component of other proteins and enzymes that are involved in the synthesis of collagen and various neurotransmitters. What is consistently and routinely lost in the world of conventional medicine is that *for iron to be functional, adequate levels of copper must be bioavailable.* This is the foundational Yin-yang of our metabolism as born out in thousands of research studies completed annually around the globe. Regrettably, these cupro-ironic insights and essentials are apparently not taught in any doctor school. Their restricted training is, indeed, iron-ic.

Hemoglobin is made up of four heme groups. Heme protein is a very foundational protein in the body but our bodies cannot make heme and knit those four heme groups together without bioavailable copper (Cartwright and Wintrobe, 1958; Ames et al, 2005). To insert the iron into each of those heme groups, which is the last of eight key enzyme steps to make heme, requires an enzyme called ferrochelatase. Ferrochelatase doesn't work without bioavailable copper. It is also worth noting that the first and last three steps of making heme proteins occurs within the mitochondrial copper matrix. Again, there is more to the story than we have been led to believe.

Another very important function in the body is to preserve the life cycle of the red blood cell. This process is managed by an enzyme called heme oxygenase-1, which is also regulated by bioavailable copper. The entire life cycle of blood and hemoglobin is dictated by bioavailable copper's ability to manage oxidative stress, but we've not been taught that. Nor is this important fact emphasized in practitioner training.

In reality, 95 percent of our daily need for iron comes from a recycling system known in the medical literature as the reticuloendothelial system (RES). I prefer to call it what it is: the iron REcycling System. And what's essential for this recycling system? Bioavailable copper! Without enough bioavailable copper, iron starts to build up inside the mitochondria and thus inside the cells, where it chokes off the mitochondria's ability to "breathe" and thus make energy (Mg-ATP). It is clearly noted and described in the accurate and responsible iron literature, largely coming out of Italy, Iran, Iraq, Ireland, Australia, Austria, Chile, and United Kingdom. Note the country missing in that list. And the KEY study that is repeatedly referenced as the origin of this copper<>iron dynamic is as follows: Hart, Steenbock, Waddell and Elvehjem, 1928, "Iron in nutrition. VII. Copper as a Supplement to Iron for Hemoglobin building in the Rat." *Jrl Biol Chem* 77: 797-812 (A noted plaque on the University of Wisconsin at Madison campus highlights the significance of this research, stating in the last sentence that it *"led to the use of copper to treat iron deficiency anemia."* It is worth noting that this plaque is made of brass, which is composed of mostly copper.)

For iron to be beneficial to health, it must be mobilized, meaning it needs to primarily be circulating in the body, instead of becoming unbound from blood and building up in tissues and organs. This is the key point that modern medicine completely misunderstands! Iron that is not regulated is not only dangerous, over time it can quite literally kill us! When iron levels appear low in the blood, the practitioner should IMMEDIATELY question the status of iron in the tissue, iron that is a part of this iron REcycling System. They never do, and it's one of the KEY reasons why fatigue is not fully understood, and why it is so pervasive throughout our society.

The Anemia Hoax

All of us are constantly exposed to iron toxicity due to the iron and other heavy metals that are so prevalent in our air, soil, and water supplies today. Eating so-called iron-enriched or fortified foods, as well as taking iron supplements, are two of the most common other causes of excessive iron buildup in the body.

Unbound iron and the buildup of iron where it does not belong in the body is completely overlooked by physicians and others who claim that anemia is due solely to a deficiency of iron. That is not the case at all, and I consider it a crime against humanity that this beLIEf is still being pushed by organized medicine. Iron levels are NOT a "fuel gauge," where simple high/low thinking is involved. They are, for a fact, more akin to "miles per gallon" where there are multiple variables and higher order thinking is required to better understand the truth of this dynamic.

The origin of this misunderstanding dates back to the 1920s. That was when researchers first started to explore the question of whether or not we had enough iron in our diet. Much of this early research involved pregnant women and the fact that a woman's hemoglobin levels actually decline as the months of pregnancy progress. That's a known fact. The technical term for it is hemodilution. It occurs because the expectant mother is providing for another life, and there's only so much hemoglobin to go around for mother and child. Based on that fact, the medical profession, as well as the League of Nations and its successor, the United Nations, and the World Health Organization (WHO) decided to push the theory that anemia is caused solely by an iron deficiency. But anemia is not an iron deficiency. It is, in fact, *iron dysregulation*. And this dysregulation is born of a deficiency of bioavailable copper, due to a lack of copper and retinol that are missing in the modern diet (Klevay LM 2000). Retinol is the animal-based form of vitamin A. (Hodges et al, 1978, "Hematopoietic Studies in Vitamin A Deficiency." *Am Jrl Clin Nutr* 31:876-885.) It turns out that retinol is what really brings the energy to the process that makes copper bioavailable, and also to the process of recycling iron for proper hemoglobin formation. Dr. Hodges' study is a true tour-de-force in the annals of iron metabolism. It is apparently nowhere to be found in any doctor school on this planet.

The earliest article that I have found that discussed the connection between retinol, iron, and the development of hemoglobin was published in 1855. It was written by a London physician named Theophilus Thompson, MD, who used cod liver oil to cure anemia during that time period. Unfortunately, a lot of that research has been lost to the ages. Besides, how many people want to go back to 1855, or would even trust that research, despite its accuracy? What is critical to understand is that there's way more to the "official" story about what actually regulates iron besides the proverbial recommendations for more iron, based on "fuel gauge" thinking.

In 1934, three physicians from the United States won the Nobel Prize for curing anemia and pernicious (B12) anemia. Their names were Drs. Whipple, Minot, and Murphy, and all three were highly-recognized MDs in their respective institutions (Hopkins and Harvard), and they all used the exact same product to solve the problem of anemia and B12 anemia. Do you want to guess what it was? *Beef liver!* And what most people don't know is that there is twice as much copper as there is iron in healthy beef liver from cattle allowed to eat their natural grass-fed diet. It is also worth noting that the liver is also the main storage site for both retinol and copper.

Thanks to the work of Drs. Hart, Thompson, Whipple, Minot, and Murphy, as well as Hodges, Semba, Nairz, Weiss, Kell, and many other luminary iron and nutritional researchers, we have documented evidence from both the 19th and 20th centuries that iron, alone, is not what cures anemia. Copper, that becomes catalyzed by retinol, becomes "bioavailable," and that is what enables iron to be "functional" inside our body and its many pathways.

Further enforcing this fact is research that was conducted in Berlin, Germany, in 1927, by the noted scientists and clinicians, Otto Warburg, PhD, MD and Hans Adolph Krebs, MD, PhD, both of whom went on to win Nobel Prizes (1931 and 1953, respectively). Krebs worked for Warburg from 1926-30, and in 1927 they conducted a fascinating experiment in which they took birds and bled them, almost to the point of death, to create the first true state of anemia in a laboratory setting (i.e., low to no iron in the blood). There was minimal iron left because the birds' blood loss was so great. Warburg and Krebs conducted this study because they were intensely studying the relationship of copper and iron, as were scores of scientists and clinicians in that era of the 1920s and 1930s.

When you deplete an animal of its blood, it's not going to have the life force needed to sustain itself. What Warburg and Krebs wanted to determine was what would happen when the birds were near empty of blood and depleted of that life force. What they were surprised to discover was that there was a three- to six-fold increase in copper protein/enzymes within the remaining blood of these birds. Under that kind of extreme, iron-depleted stress, the birds responded by creating copper protein/enzymes to activate the process needed to make new blood in order to compensate for this massive loss of iron. (Please take a moment to reflect on the significance of this response.) These metabolic truths are, again, not taught in doctor school. Don't be offended by the date of this research. Be in awe of the two geniuses who designed and executed this pioneering and penetrating research to reveal the truth of our physiology.

This was the exact **opposite** outcome of what they had expected, and their findings, which they published in that same year—I accessed the original version written in German and had it translated so that I could read it—led to an extensive series of further studies all over the globe about this fascinating and dynamic copper<>iron relationship.

As you consider the results of this bird experiment by Warburg and Krebs, remember the 9,000 or so enzymes that I mentioned earlier. Enzymes are what enable all of the body's chemical reactions to proceed. Without enzymes, iron cannot be incorporated into hemoglobin, and these enzymes need copper to function properly. Many of the key enzymes that are needed for the production of red blood cells and hemoglobin are copper dependent, especially those needed to make energy (cytochrome c oxidase) and to clear exhaust (SOD, glutathione peroxidase or catalase). That is why the copper protein/enzymes increased so much in those birds that were bled down. The birds needed to get more of the copper protein/enzymes functioning in order to utilize the raw material (iron) that was remaining there.

In the same way, if someone is anemic, meaning that iron is not in the blood, it is more than likely due to a lack of bioavailable copper. The iron is not attached to hemoglobin in the blood where it belongs, it is immobilized in the tissues and unable to be properly released to the REcycling System and brought to the bone marrow where iron is then incorporated into 2-3 million RBC precursor cells made each and every second.

The body has three requirements to make blood. First, it has to be able to produce energy. Second, it has to able to make iron sulfur clusters, which are found all over the body. And third, it has to be able to make heme, which are based on iron sulfur clusters. But the body cannot make energy, iron sulfur clusters, or heme, without bioavailable copper. In 1939, M.O. Schultze, PhD, added an additional requirement: The need for the key antioxidant enzyme, catalase, which maintains equilibrium in the cells and in the blood, and has a dependence on copper. These facts are clearly spelled out in the medical literature, yet it is still not common knowledge, not just among the public, but among most practitioners! Since doctors don't know these central copper facts, they continue to regard anemia as solely an "iron deficiency" problem, and completely overlook the body of research and literature that has focused on copper deficiency anemia since the 1950s. At the same time, many of these same doctors warn their patients that copper is toxic. I cannot stress this point enough:

Copper is not toxic and iron is not deficient.

(Please take another moment to re-read that sentence, again. Now, pause and reflect on what that might mean for you if you've been told that you are anemic, and if you have struggled with fatigue for any length of time.) Could Mark Twain, in fact, be right?

For most people today, copper is, in fact, missing in action because we don't have enough of it, and iron, rather than being deficient, is stuck ("dysfunctional") in our tissues. Again, it is this lack of bioavailable copper that causes iron to become stuck and accumulate where it does not belong, especially in cells called "recycling macrophages" that are key to proper iron recycling and healthy copper<>iron metabolism.

Returning to how the body produces heme, at the end of that process there are eight enzymes that are involved. Four of them are active outside of the mitochondria, and four of them perform their tasks inside the mitochondrial copper matrix. The four inside the mitochondria all require copper, and the last one is the most important as we've discussed previously.

Ferrochelatase acts like a crane. And that crane operator is a copper ion that directs the acquisition of the iron needed and drops it into the center of the heme molecule. If you don't have that cupro-crane operator, the iron doesn't get dropped into heme, and then the body then can't produce hemoglobin naturally or efficiently. And to broaden our awareness of these dynamics, there is an enormous amount of heme, hemoglobin and erythrocytes (RBCs) made daily:

- 2-3 million RBCs are made every second, thus >200 billion every 24 hours
- There are ~270 million hemoglobin in each RBC
- There are 4 heme inside each hemoglobin
- There are ~1 billion heme in each RBC

You can quickly see the enormous demands for not just iron, but also for bioavailable copper. It is high time the world awaken to this critical need for the catalytic and regulatory requirements that only bioavailable copper facilitates within our metabolism and within our mitochondria! What is sobering to learn is that these Cupro-truths about the essential role for copper to ensure functional iron have been known since the 1920's worldwide (McHargue, 1925; Hart et al, 1928; Elvehjem, 1929; Underwood, 1935).

Most doctors interpret the problem of insufficient hemoglobin to mean their patients have a lack of sufficient iron. They assume that because the crane operator (copper) wasn't there, it must mean that there isn't enough needed iron. That is absolutely not true. In fact, it is just the opposite. Another important point that practitioners seem to overlook is that bioavailable copper needs to be expressed via its enzymes, especially ferroxidase, its principal antioxidant enzyme. Ferroxidase was discovered in 1948 by two Swedish physiologists, Carl G. Holmberg and C.B Laurell, and when discovered, they thought they had discovered the holy grail. As we've explored, ferroxidase is able to work with iron in the presence of oxygen, without giving off any reactive oxygen species or oxidants. It is the master antioxidant enzyme that regulates iron status in the body. It is also one aspect of the active form of ceruloplasmin, and in this capacity it prevents iron from "rusting"/oxidizing, and, just as importantly, regulates and manages the movement of iron from tissue to blood, where iron belongs, and so that it can return to the bone marrow where it is regularly and routinely recycled back into new red blood cells.

Again, over 200 billion red blood cells are produced every 24 hours.

There are eight copper atoms that power the ferroxidase enzymes. 95 percent of serum copper is designed to be complexed inside of ceruloplasmin. Ferroxidase is a very important enzyme, considered by many scientists to be the master antioxidant protein/enzyme in the human body. When our bodies have abundant sources of it, iron is kept in proper regulation and proper homeostasis. Iron homeostasis is like a seesaw. On one end is iron in the blood. On the other end is iron in the tissue, and the fulcrum managing this critical balance is the ferroxidase enzyme making sure that the ferroportin (FPN) doorway is open and regularly releasing iron to our transferrin proteins. Because doctors are not taught about the role and importance of ferroxidase enzyme, they are prone to interpret "low iron in the blood" as the sole reason for anemia, and then tell their patients they are "anemic" because they were not completely trained about the central role of ferroxidase in this critical seesaw process of iron homeostasis.

Ceruloplasmin, acting through its ferroxidase enzyme, plays a pivotal role in keeping this iron-ic "seesaw" in balance to maintain proper iron metabolism and homeostasis, while also protecting against oxidation by converting toxic ferrous (Fe++) iron into its nontoxic ferric (Fe+++) form that can bind with proteins. The ferroxidase activity of ceruloplasmin is what helps keep iron mobilized so that it does not allow iron to get stuck in the tissue. This being so, it should be obvious by now that lack of ceruloplasmin/ferroxidase activity is intimately responsible for what is mistakenly (myth-takenly) being diagnosed as "anemia." And entirely missing in this process is any effective or convenient way to measure iron status *inside our tissues.*

What is central to understanding this key distinction is to not misdiagnose the problem as "*iron deficiency,*" when the blood problem is the result of "*iron dysregulation,*" for lack of sufficient bioavailable copper. It is this latter situation that is known as "anemia of chronic disease," and "anemia of chronic inflammation" that is known in research circles to be caused by a lack of bioavailable copper. (Cartwright GE and Wintrobe MM, 1952, The Anemia of Infection. XVII. *A Review in Advances in Internal Medicine,* Dock W & Snapper I, Eds, Chicago, Year Book Publishers; Vol 5, Pg 165.)

More About "Anemia" That Your Doctor Doesn't Emphasize

Here are some more facts to explain why I consider iron deficiency anemia to be one of the biggest myths on this planet:

- 70 percent of the iron in our body is found in the hemoglobin of our red blood cells. There needs to be lots of magnesium in the red blood cells in order to make energy so that the red blood cells can live a full life (optimal lifespan of healthy red blood cells is~120 days), and remain flexible, pliable and able to get into tight spaces. If red blood cells can't do that, then we've got a problem. When there is either a magnesium or a copper deficiency, the RBC lifespan can drop to as little as 20 days. That is an extraordinary loss (80%) of lifespan. Doctors regularly mistake this problem to be yet another sign of anemia.

- Red blood cells float in an extracellular medium called plasma, which has essentially the mineral composition of sea water, but contains less sodium (Na). This plasma contains many minerals, including copper, in order to be healthy and to clear the exhaust that occurs within and outside of these red blood cells. One of the most important antioxidant enzymes in our body is SOD-1 (copper/zinc superoxide dismutase-1), which exists to combat the oxidative stress that naturally occurs inside the red blood cells. There is another important anti-oxidant enzyme, SOD-3, (extracellular or erythrocyte superoxide dismutase-3) to combat oxidative stress in the plasma that is OUTSIDE the RBCs, which is why it's called "extracellular." These enzymes are essential because of the RBCs' high oxygen and high iron content. There need to be mechanisms to clear that oxidative exhaust because it's a natural process of breakdown that occurs routinely within our blood. Without copper, this breakdown leads to added oxidative stress that causes energy loss that has nothing whatsoever to do with a lack of iron.

- There are different ways in which what is called anemia can occur. One of the main ways has to do with iron in the gut not being able to be delivered into the bloodstream. This occurs when iron in the gut cannot pass out of the enterocytes, the first line of cells in the digestive tract. Central to this understanding is knowing how iron gets absorbed into our gut and then released into our blood stream. The process of iron absorption in the digestive tract has two steps. The first step involves getting iron *into the enterocytes* (the cells that line our digestive tract), which occurs fairly easily. The rate of absorption varies based on whether it is heme iron, which has an absorption rate of approximately 40 percent, or non-heme iron from grains and vegetables, which has an absorption rate of between 15 and 20 percent. However, the inorganic iron filings being added to wheat flour is estimated to have a higher absorption rate of~60 percent, which is an absolute abomination to our digestive tract.

The second step—moving iron *out of the enterocytes and into the bloodstream*—is where the real challenge occurs. For this to happen, iron must pass through that ferroportin (FPN) doorway. As we've noted, this passage requires bioavailable copper expressing as the ferroxidase enzyme to 1) facilitate the release of iron, 2) the opening of the doorway AND 3) the incorporation of iron onto the transport protein, transferrin. When ferroxidase enzyme is present and active, the exiting iron can then be safely and properly loaded onto transferrin so that the iron can make its way to either the bone marrow for new blood formation or to the liver for storage and use at a later time. It is worth noting that these two proteins, ceruloplasmin and transferrin, represent a critical portion of the body's innate immune system, which is designed to keep iron in the blood ***properly bound*** and ***properly circulating***. Otherwise, pathogens will hijack that iron and use it to run their own replication machinery.

Without copper and the ferroxidase enzyme activity, iron delivery into the bloodstream is greatly impaired. Enough iron is still in the body, but it is not getting out of the digestive tissue (enterocytes) and not getting into the bloodstream to be transported where it belongs principally. Again, this inadequate movement of iron has nothing whatsoever to do with a deficiency of iron. It is the epitome of iron dysregulation caused by a lack of bioavailable copper.

As an important aside, it is important to also know that calcitriol, the active form of what is mistakenly referred to as vitamin D (in reality, it's a hormone), has the unique ability to increase the synthesis of nitric oxide, which then opens the FPN doorway without the presence of copper to allow unregulated iron out. This can be a "D"isaster, and the average doctor has no awareness as to why this is an issue that can trigger what is commonly known as "leaky gut syndrome," causing a metabolic crisis. In Chapter 9, I explain, in detail, why vitamin D supplements are also dangerous to your health, contrary to what you might think or have been trained to beLIEve.

Another form of anemia occurs from restricted iron delivery in the spleen. This happens when the spleen can't clear what are called red pulp macrophages (RPMs). RPMs are necessary for red blood cell homeostasis and thus critical for iron recycling. If the RPMs cannot turn over the red blood cells, then iron cannot be returned back to the bone marrow to make new red blood cells. This condition is known as sideroblastic, or sideroachrestic, anemia, a type of anemia in which the bone marrow produces "ringed sideroblasts" rather than healthy red blood cells, in large part because the forming RBCs are not able to release their iron due to a dysfunction of the copper-dependent ferroportin doorway (noted above) not being able to work properly in these maturing red blood cells. The body has plenty of iron available, but once again cannot release it to then incorporate it into hemoglobin, which red blood cells need in order to transport oxygen efficiently.

Hemoglobin is heme plus globulin (alpha globulins and beta globulins).If you can't make globulin, you can't make hemoglobin. It turns out that all four of these components require copper. Again, this mineral foundation is not taught to practitioners, but if iron can't get out of the gut and can't recycle properly in the spleen, and if the heme can't be made in the bone marrow, the result is merely different forms of anemia, *but they all originate from a lack of bioavailable copper, not from a lack of iron.* But what's the number one "solution" for all of these issues that doctors consistently recommend? ***Add more iron!*** And that, in my humble opinion, is where the crisis of fatigue really begins. People keep getting drowned in iron when in fact what they simply need is more bioavailable copper, but that mineral reality is well outside the training of most health practitioners. Maybe this book can serve to pique their curiosity to what else might cause this iron-ic dynamic in their patients' symptoms.

We have a lot of iron dysfunction because there isn't enough bioactive copper. It is not a deficiency of iron. Yet when was the last time your doctor measured your serum copper (ideal = 100), your serum ceruloplasmin (ideal = 30), or computed your copper/ceruloplasmin ratio, which should be 3.33 (Scheinberg IH and Sternlieb I, 1960)?

What is useful to understand is that under conditions of what the immune system perceives as chronic disease or chronic inflammation, our macrophages are called upon to increase the production and release of a key molecule called nitric oxide (NO*). It is an ancient molecule on this planet and scientists refer to it as the smallest hormone in our body. Among its many jobs is to activate the body's innate immune system. Under these conditions, NO* naturally blocks the actions of the first and eighth (last) enzymes in the production of heme. Because there is no regular nor routine assessment of NO* status, doctors mistake the low hemoglobin as a sign of low iron, and not high inflammation. (Weiss G, 1999; Weiss G and Goodnough LT, 2005; Nairz M, Weiss G et al, 2014)

Again, think about the amount of heme needed per second. In addition, there is supposed to be ferritin (a storage protein for iron) inside the mitochondria to gobble up this iron, but that iron loading function also requires bioavailable copper, otherwise known as ceruloplasmin. And finally, there is also supposed to be superoxide dismutase. Superoxide is regularly being formed at Complex I and Complex III of the mitochondrial ETC (electron transport chain) that we discussed in Chapter 3, and it is also reacting with iron. Superoxide dismutase (SOD-1 and SOD-3) require copper, as well. When we're missing the copper in these critical areas, hemoglobin production will and does fall off.

Has your doctor ever taught you ANY of this? Not likely. In fairness, most doctors were never taught these details outlined above. Instead, when they see low iron markers in the blood, they are NOT trained to question iron in the tissue versus iron in the blood, and automatically think "iron deficiency anemia." The truth of the matter, as you know by now, is that the "deficiency" is actually a dysfunction. It is a lack of functional iron. Always remember: There is a big difference between iron in the blood versus iron in the tissue. And where there is dysfunctional iron, there is sure to be a lack of bioavailable copper and a corresponding gain of oxidative stress. Again, this is not my idea. Please understand that these concepts are not my "opinion." They are a "compendium" and a synthesis of hundreds of scientific studies on copper-iron metabolism that I've had the benefit of reading this past decade. These many articles form a mineral-based tapestry to redefine how energy is made and how energy is lost within the human organism, and ultimately, how these dynamics affect copper<>iron metabolism.

These energy problems exist because of a lack of bioavailable copper. That is what is lost on conventional practitioners of all faiths and persuasions. They are blind to the difference between iron in the blood and iron in the tissue, as well as the role of ferroxidase as the seesaw regulating the flow of iron between these two settings. Again, it is bioavailable copper that allows iron to get out of the tissue and get back into the bloodstream so that it can be part of this vital, daily iron REcycling System, aka RES (reticuloendothelial system). Our bodies need a turnover of iron every 24 hours. One percent of our RBCs die each day and need to be replaced. Key to this entire process is that ceruloplasmin (via ferroxidase function) increases the rate of iron release by two and a half times (Sarkar J, Fox PL et al, 2003-Nov7, "Role of Cp with Macrophage Iron Efflux During Hypoxia" *Jrl Biol Chem* 275(45): 44018-44024). This accelerated iron release is a central biological mechanism that is clearly not taught in any doctor school. I'm hoping that this book, along with the research highlighted, will inspire a change in that contemporary educational and clinical gap.

Furthermore, an important study by Killilea and Ames (2004) demonstrated that iron in the tissue (fibroblasts) can be as much as ten times higher than iron in the blood. This is a watershed study that challenges the conventional narrative of "iron deficiency." What is missing in all this confusion is that there is no simple, nor painless test for measuring iron in the tissue, other than a needle biopsy of the liver or a T2 MRI of the organs. Again, please know that the blood test of iron has no relevance to iron status *in the tissue*. They are completely different media and need to be understood and treated as such. (Note: pies on the counter do not equal pies in the oven...)

All practitioners know about is iron in the blood, because they don't know what they don't know. And they don't know what they don't look for. They believe that iron is low in the blood, and therefore their patient's needs more iron. People keep getting supplemented and infused with iron when in fact what they need is more bioavailable copper. *That is why I keep saying that missing information equals missing TRUTH.* When a cow is not producing milk, do farmers correct that cow's problem? Or do they just keep adding more cows to the herd? Farmers know that they need to solve the problem, not keep adding to their expenses with additional cows. But it seems that practitioners are trained to only keep adding more iron to the problem without correcting the underlying cause of the "low iron in the blood."

How Standard Iron Tests Make Matters Worse

Standard iron tests today typically include measuring iron levels in the blood (hemoglobin, serum iron and serum ferritin). If any of these tests show low levels of iron in the blood, doctors tell their patients they are anemic. That's a problem, and another example of how poorly trained doctors are about iron metabolism and the roles of bioavailable copper to ensure iron homeostasis. Again, they make no distinction between iron in the blood versus iron in the tissue. And as noted above, iron levels in the tissue can be ten times higher than that in the blood. Additionally, ferritin, which is an iron storage protein, is supposed to be inside of our cells in the tissues of the body, not found in our blood, which flows outside of our cells.

Here are the key points you need to remember:

Low levels of iron in the blood do not mean low iron levels in the tissue of our body. It more than likely means that iron is stuck in the tissues because it is not being properly mobilized due to lack of bioavailable copper, best expressed through the ferroxidase enzyme.

Doctors don't say a word to their patients about oxygen and oxidative stress that exists in the body, and which are aggravated by added iron. And there is not one word about copper, and its known properties and abilities to harness and regulate two very reactive elements in our body: *oxygen* and *iron*. Copper stands alone in its unique ability to harness oxygen and regulate iron. Call me crazy, but I think those are very important concepts for people, including their practitioners, to know and properly understand. Again, missing information equals missing truth.

Another important nuance of this dynamic is to understand how the focus on ferritin began in 1972, when a British team of researchers published an article that put the spotlight on this iron storage protein (Jacobs A et al, 1972, "Ferritin in the Serum of Normal Subjects and Patients with Iron Deficiency and Iron Overload." *Br Med Jrl* 4: 206-208). In the tissues of the body there is ferritin (in the cells) and mito-ferritin (in the mitochondria), which are both found inside the cells. They act as storage lockers for iron. Beyond this, it is important to understand that there are really three forms of ferritin: heavy chain (which requires ferroxidase enzyme function to load iron into it), light chain (that acts independent of the enzyme) and serum ferritin that is an abridged form of light chain ferritin, is actually empty of iron, and is being excreted into the serum as a sign of inflammation (Kell DB and Pretorius E, 2010). Serum ferritin is not a measure of intracellular ferritin. It is a blood test that is measuring an altered ferritin protein showing up in the extracellular medium of the blood, and that blood is outside of the cell. Yes, this is wildly confusing. I have renamed this iron storage marker "***Errortin***" as it is entirely deceptive and misrepresents true iron status in our body.

Intracellular ferritin represents less than ten percent of the iron in the body—in some research studies, I've seen it as low as one percent—as opposed to the 70 percent of body iron that hemoglobin represents. Doctors are routinely measuring an intracellular protein (ferritin) in an extracellular medium (blood). This is akin to measuring hay in a barn versus hay in the field. If you want to know how many bales of hay you have in the barn, you do not go outside into the field to start counting it. That simply does NOT make any sense, and neither does measuring ferritin outside of the cell, when it belongs and is metabolically designed to be inside the cells.

In addition, there is the difference between ferritin and hemosiderin to be considered. Hemosiderin is an additional iron storage complex when cellular iron status becomes excessive. When intracellular ferritin becomes "denatured," it becomes hemosiderin. What is important to understand is that ***hemosiderin can house up to ten times more iron than ferritin***. Again, iron is not candy. It is the master prooxidant element on the planet. Now here's the kicker: When was the last time your doctor measured your hemosiderin level? Never, right? If you have a pulse, your spider sense should be quivering right about now, especially if you've been told *"You're anemic!"* If you are or have been taking iron supplements for any extended period of time, this should challenge your perception that you're anemic. Again, persistent use of supplemental iron will never correct the copper deficiency that's causing your iron to appear "low" in the blood, even though you may have notable pockets of hemosiderin. (Not known, because not looked for is the mantra of medicine.)

Another important point to remember is that blood is, in essence, a transport medium. Blood has to stay at a very specific pH of about 7.4. If it varies too much below or above that, we die. In order to maintain that pH level, the body moves minerals in and out of the blood. Trying to assume that a blood level of iron (or any other substance) is the same thing as an iron tissue level is simply not correct for this reason.

As my friend and colleague Ben Edwards, MD points out, thyroid hormone is a great example of this. *"The amount of thyroid hormone in your blood may not necessarily correlate with what's in the cell,"* he notes. *"The thyroid hormone in the blood is T4 but T3 is what's needed inside the cell, and the body has a process to get it into the cell where it can go do its job. Measuring what's in the blood doesn't tell you what's inside the cell. We've got to be careful and we've got to have a deeper understanding of physiology and blood work and what the blood work is really showing us."*

Most doctors recognize and accept what Ben says about thyroid hormones, yet they remain blind to the exact same dynamic that is involved with ferritin and iron in the blood as opposed to what is inside the cells. As a result, they continue to myth-diagnose "anemia" because they focus on ferritin and serum iron levels while bypassing the broader complexity of the iron REcycling System and overall iron homeostasis. And, because of their scripted training, they pay no attention whatsoever to copper, ceruloplasmin, especially its ferroxidase enzyme activity, with its eight copper atoms that enables iron to move from tissue to blood faster, thus falsely insisting that low serum iron levels mean that patients have an iron deficiency. The real problem is that the iron is physiologically prevented from moving into the blood due to the lack of ferroxidase activity at the FPN (ferroportin) doorway. They are not measuring iron in the tissue because they were not trained completely to understand these many nuances of copper-iron metabolism.

The entire body of practitioners worldwide operates from this dangerous narrow-minded training. Adding insult to this clinical misunderstanding, for nearly a century, in the US, UK, Canada, and the developing countries that they feed, there has been the fortification of their foods with nine different forms of iron. Given what we are learning here, this added iron may be to the added detriment of our health.

Having read this far, you now know how and why excess iron can become dysregulated, meaning unable to be mobilized from tissues into the blood, which triggers destructive oxidation as oxygen reacts with it. I would contend that this growing dysregulation between missing copper and fortified iron is the real metabolic cause of chronic fatigue that leads to the inevitable chronic conditions that now dominate a once healthy society. Regrettably, and iron-ically, this is not rocket science, but it does involve being open to NEW incorporations of OLD and ENDURING copper<>iron research.

A fundamental paradigm of the Root Cause Protocol is that as we age, we lose copper. That is an established biological fact, and copper is key to harnessing oxygen and iron. Every day of our lives, iron is building up in our bodies at the rate of a milligram a day (private conversation with Robert R. Crichton, PhD, world renowned iron expert), and the oxidants that are also created in our bodies each day release catalytic iron in its ferrous ($Fe++$) form. It is ferrous iron that donates an electron in a reaction with hydrogen peroxide to generate the hydroxyl radical, a violently reactive oxygen species (ROS), causing oxidative stress, lipid peroxidation, and DNA damage, and thus metabolic breakdown that inevitably leads to fatigue and chronic conditions (Fenton HJH, 1894).

Over time, as ferrous iron continues to build up, it is stored, first and foremost, in the liver, which, when we are young, ideally starts out in a normal, healthy state, but then, becomes what I refer to as a "ferrous wheel" as it takes on more and more of this heavy metal. Doctors and other health practitioners are taught to "treat the seats" of this ferrous wheel. And in like fashion, they are taught and trained to ignore the axle of mineral and metabolic dysfunction, which is the entire focus of the Root Cause Protocol and why it has immediate, metabolic impact.

Imagine an actual Ferris wheel with its outer circle of seats, all connected by spokes to the wheel's center, or hub. The seats are the secondary effects, or symptoms, of the actual underlying dysregulation (disease) originating at the hub. All that doctors are taught to do for their patients is to treat the seats (symptoms), without paying any attention to the actual root causes that are unfolding in the hub. They overlook the increasing iron dysregulation and the corresponding oxidative stress that follows. *This is why fatigue persistently remains their patients' most common health complaint*, and is also why over 85 percent of all conditions today are considered "chronic." These severe problems, which cost our nation over three trillion dollars a year in so-called "healthcare" expenditures, will never be solved by conventional medicine's current paradigm because doctors are trained to only focus on and attempt to manage symptoms.

By contrast, the Root Cause Protocol is focused on correcting the core hub of the problem by bringing copper, magnesium, other key minerals and vitamin complexes into alignment with proper regulation and management of iron and oxygen. Through the use of nutrient dense foods and necessary nutritional supplements we have designed an easy to adopt protocol that solves the redox cycling pathology initiated by unchecked oxidative stress that is the underlying cause of all fatigue that then ushers in all known chronic conditions. That is why the Root Cause Protocol works so well for the thousands of people around the world who have put it into practice, and why it can work so well for you, too.

Know The Cause and Address It

"Destiny in not a matter of chance. It is a matter of choice. It is not a thing to be waited for. It is a thing to be achieved."
– William Jennings Bryan

"In the middle of every difficulty lies opportunity"
– Albert Einstein

Congratulations!

Now that you've read this far, you have a deeper and more accurate understanding of the true metabolic root causes of both fatigue and disease These are concepts that I'm confident our doctors would enjoy learning were it made a formal part of their curriculum. I realize that may sound optimistic, but we've got to start this dialogue somewhere, so it might as well be this book.

What you learned in the previous chapters, especially the information in Chapters 3 and 4, is simply not taught in doctor schools, even though the science clearly supports all that I have shared with you thus far. This is true not only of mainstream, conventional medical schools, but also of institutions and organizations focused on providing training in integrative, functional, naturopathic, alternative, nutritional, and orthomolecular medicine. The sad truth is that practitioners in all of these fields rarely, if ever, go beyond the training and formal education they received. Therefore, they can only reply upon what they have been taught, virtually none of which explains or addresses the actual underlying metabolic dynamics, which are the most basic reasons why their patients are tired and unhealthy.

Moreover, what these doctors and other health practitioners have been taught can, and often does, make their patients' metabolic conditions worse. This includes their conventional nutritional recommendations, if the physicians even give a moment's consideration to their patients' diet and any nutritional supplements they might be taking. The vast majority of conventional MDs ignore this most important foundation of health altogether. How can they do otherwise, when they have had virtually no training in it? That is a fact, as Ben Edwards, MD, confirmed in this book's Introduction, pointing out how little, to no, education he and other medical students receive related to diet and nutrition, in general and mineral metabolism, in particular. This is a well-known educational gap in conventional medical training.

Even the recommendations provided to patients by so-called nutritionally oriented health care practitioners who do focus on this area can also be harmful and perpetuate illness and fatigue. This is particularly true of their recommendation to take synthetic vitamins C and D, both of which, as you will discover in Chapter 9 do the exact opposite of what they are claimed to do. Instead of supporting health, these substances severely and negatively limit the amount of bioavailable copper that you now know is the key nutrient, along with magnesium and real vitamin A (retinol), that you most need for optimal energy and good health. Recommendations to supplement with other nutrients, such as calcium and zinc, are also challenging, as Chapter 8 explains. And, of course, as you now understand, iron supplements intended to "correct" the chronically incorrect diagnoses of anemia can be incredibly dysruptive, as well.

So what is the solution to this mass epidemic of nutritional distortion among doctors and other practitioners in the so-called health care field? Since we can't seem to rely on these "experts," what can we do?

To me, there is only one worthwhile and effective answer to these critical questions. We need to become our own health expert and be willing to experiment in and on our own God-given laboratory— our body.

Central to this process is a willingness to step outside the box of conventional, mainstream "expert" advice—both from modern medicine and from our government agencies at the local, state, and federal levels— that has been directly responsible for turning the United States into the sickest industrialized nation on the planet, costing us nearly $3.5 trillion each year to boot. Please keep in mind, that before the advent of World War II, the United States was considered the healthiest country in the world. Now 80 years later, we are hovering near the bottom! That is quite an alarming drop in just three generations. Instead, we need to discover for ourselves what actually works to improve our energy, and thus our health, and what does not. Just as I had to do for my own health and well-being. Just as thousands of other people, just like you, have done once they began to adopt and work with the nutrients emphasized in the Root Cause Protocol.

In the previous chapters, you learned the most essential and foundational principles that optimal health depends upon. When those principles are violated or ignored, energy loss leads to fatigue which directly leads to metabolic dysfunction, which then leads to the prevalence of symptoms that eventually leads to a "disease process" that inevitably and inexorably will follow. When this happens, practitioners resort to "labeling" their patients with a specific disease category: Alzheimer's, arthritis, chronic fatigue, cancer, diabetes, heart disease, MS, Parkinson's, irritable bowel syndrome, and on and on.

The names and these diagnoses do not matter. What does matter is that America today is chronically ill and has been for decades precisely because the foundational principles of health are being overlooked and compromised. Not only by the public at large and their practitioners, but also by and because of the pharmaceutical industry, the monopoly cartels of Big Agriculture, Big Chemical, Big Hospital, and various other special interest sectors, all of which have their paws and beaks deep in the multitrillion dollar trough that Big Disease generates each and every year. I know this well as I was a part of that industry for 32 years. I know the belly of this beast.

Disease diagnoses are made by physicians because they are not trained to recognize and understand the underlying mineral dysregulation that causes metabolic dysfunction that is the real underlying issue, and which then causes oxidative stress, the underlying catalyst for all symptoms. How these imbalances manifest depend on each person's individual degree of chronic stress, their diet, their environment, their mineral composition, and various other factors. Genes are also a factor, but genes are ruled by epigenetics (the environment in which genes find themselves) and our epigenetics are ultimately ruled by our mitochondrial energetics. For some people, the imbalances may lead to diabetes; for others, perhaps heart disease or cancer. A major contributing factor is the underlying stress and emotions that they are chronically experiencing.

However these mineral and metabolic imbalances manifest as a health issue, the symptoms themselves are a downstream effect of these imbalances. This is very important for us to realize.

If we are suffering from fatigue and/or chronic illness, we cannot, and will not, get better if we focus on treating these effects, which are essentially all that mainstream medicine does. Not understanding or overlooking the actual root cause of the health problems their patients are experiencing results in most doctors resorting to merely managing symptoms, which is why the majority of their patients remain fatigued and chronically unwell. You might have picked up this book because you are one of those patients and are desperate for new information so that you can select a better and more fundamental path for recovery. Well, I can assure you that you've found it. Now all you have to do is apply it– with patience, persistence, and confidence!

Healing By Unlearning

When I began my own healing journey, I soon discovered that most of what I had learned about what it takes to become and stay healthy was incomplete and simply wrong as it was not centered on the downstream impact of energy deficiency. Dangerously so. As I shared in Chapter 1, I even considered chiropractic care to be "witchcraft" and at first stubbornly refused to try it when I suffered mightily with that frozen shoulder. I thought I was right because at the time I still believed, and was immersed, in conventional thinking and treatments.

The truth, however, was that much of what I believed to be "factual" and "evidenced-based" was incomplete. It was little more than a collection of packaged concepts that had been handed down to me—and very likely to you, as well—which I had accepted at face value, without question. In short, I had been programmed to think about disease, but not about energy.

It was only after I reached the point that my shoulder pain and limited range of motion became so intolerable to me that I finally relented and agreed to a series of chiropractic treatments. Between the chiropractic sessions and my "discovery" of magnesium, which I began to supplement with, my shoulder was soon pain-free and its full range of motion restored within a matter of weeks. I was astonished by how rapidly I healed.

It was this experience that changed my life forever, causing me to reexamine everything I thought I knew about health and healing. Up until that point, I had thought I knew quite a lot. After all, I was a hospital executive and had even studied "pre-med" while in college. What I have since discovered was that I knew very little. As I said, I had simply been programmed to think I knew the answer. Now, over a decade into this "unlearning and relearning" process, I'm simply amazed at what I've learned, but also at how much more there is to learn.

One of my favorite quotations comes from the famous author and diarist Anäis Nin, who observed, *"We don't see things as they are. We see them as we are."* I wholeheartedly agree. How we see things is a function of our experiences, our perceptions, and our beliefs. That is why, when we encounter ideas and concepts that run counter to what we believe and think we know, we run the risk of automatically rejecting them without taking the time to examine if they might contain something of value that can actually help us. That is what I initially did when chiropractic care was suggested as a possible solution for my shoulder pain. I was that cynic that Ben Edwards, MD talks about. I have since learned to be a more of a skeptic and rely upon scientific research to soothe and resolve my skepticism.

Resisting new ideas and concepts that seem to threaten our long-held, even cherished, beliefs is part of our shared human nature, unfortunately. But, as the saying goes, insanity is doing the same thing over and over again and expecting a different result. If you are always tired, or struggling with a chronic health issue, it should be obvious that whatever you have been doing to alleviate your problem is not working. You need to confront that truth, accept it and be willing to let go of the concepts and recommendations that you have been given by your doctor and others that have not provided you with the relief you are looking for.

This process of doing so is sometimes referred to as unlearning, meaning letting go of what we think we know and have been taught so that we create the space and the opportunity for ourselves to discover what actually is true and does work. That is what the Root Cause Protocol is designed to do for you. As you apply its principles to your life, they will begin to change who you are, and what you see, and what your perception and beliefs are. Particularly with regard to the minerals that we've discussed in the previous chapters and how they affect your health and overall well-being.

Until now, you have most likely relied upon your doctor or other health practitioner to help you, with little to show for it, otherwise you probably would not be reading this book. Just as Dorothy in *The Wizard of Oz* was looking for way to get back home, you have been looking for the way back to good health and lasting energy.

One of my favorite scenes in *The Wizard of Oz* is when the wizard is exposed by none other than Toto as he instructs Dorothy to pay no attention to the man behind the green curtain. But it's too late. Toto pulls the curtain back and the great and mysterious Oz is revealed to be just a man pretending to be more than he was behind the curtain. In many ways, the wizard is like modern practitioners today. That said, think of me as Toto, if you will, exposing that there's more to the story than what people have been led to believe. I think it's time for all of us to come to that critical realization. It's very important that we realize that we do need to make a change in how we see things so that we can improve not only our health, but the health of the entire planet. That is the choice we are all being presented with now. As highlighted in the opening quotations, our lives and our fate are a tapestry of the choices that we've made day-by-day. I'm inviting you to make some new choices that I'm confident will stimulate your energy production and your improved health.

I urge you to contemplate that statement because the destiny of your health and your future truly is in your control, not in the hands and whims of fate. That fact, and the importance of conscious choice, was first driven home to me when I was 31 years old and attended a weekend seminar presented by another famous speaker and motivational coach, Lou Tice, the founder of the Pacific Institute, which is dedicated to helping individuals and organizations discover and unleash their full potential. I remember that training like it happened yesterday. It was one of the most powerful experiences in my life. It changed my worldview, and because of it, ever since I have understood how important our choices are, each and every day.

Lou began his career as a high school football coach and he relished finding ways to bring out the best in people. Two of Lou's most famous sayings are, "Life is about choices, and you have the ability to choose. You always have had this ability. I suggest that not only do you have the ability, you have the responsibility to make choices for yourself. It is your life, and you are in the driver's seat, if you choose to be." And my favorite, "All meaningful and lasting change starts from the inside."

Lou's overriding message was that there's only one thing we have to do in life. We have to die. *Everything else is a choice.* He advised doing things because you want to, you choose to, you like it, or you love it. versus because you *have to.* ("Have to" is the wording of a victim.) This quote is one of my lifelong guiding aphorisms. Our lives and our fate are a tapestry of the choices that we've made day-by-day.

Operating from conscious choice because you want to do so versus making decisions because you feel you have to, which is no real choice at all, is a very powerful and empowering shift. I encourage each person reading this book to take the time to reflect on this invitation.

What I listen for when I'm doing a consultation or talking with friends and family is how many times I hear them say, *"I have to"* about this or that. For example, I'd love to take a vacation but I have to stay home because I'm always so tired and don't have the energy to do things. I tell them that every time they say and believe statements like that they are acting like a victim. And there is no reason for it. We are always free to choose something different and better. An important axiom, our words become our world.

I point this out to clients all the time. One of the most powerful parts of our dialogue is when they realize that they do have a choice. Even the illnesses that people have that seem overwhelming are not being done *to them*, they are being done *for them*. They are opportunities to learn how to grow, to really go within and reflect about what they can learn from these challenging experiences. Once they shift their focus on learning the lessons within their experiences, shifts and in some cases, miracles, start to happen. They get to the bottom of their problems, discover new ways of solving them, and get better. I am living proof of that, and so are the thousands of people who have already restored their health by following the Root Cause Protocol.

Now it's your turn to do the same!

The Next Step

The preceding chapters provided you with all the information you need to understand how and why fatigue and symptoms and eventual disease occurs in the body, as well as what you can and need to do in order to maintain and improve your energy levels and reverse any other health challenges you may currently be facing. Your next step is to learn each of the STOPS and the STARTS of the Root Cause Protocol so that you can begin to apply them. The chapters that follow in Part Two will supply you with all of the information you need in order to do so. Once you learn and understand this information, it will up to you to put it to work for you. Again, the choice is yours.

As you begin your new health journey using the Root Cause Protocol, there is one more very important piece of information you need to understand and internalize. When it comes to you and your health, there is only one true expert on whom you can always rely. That expert is not me, it is not your doctor, it is not a health organization, a health website, or anyone or anything else.

That expert is you!

What I mean by this is that you know yourself, your body, your energy levels, and how you feel overall far better and more clearly than anyone else possibly can. Because this is so, I encourage you to take what you learn in the chapters in Part Two and truly put it to the test. The RCP is designed to give you a comprehensive framework of principles and how-to instructions that you can experiment with and adapt to while always heeding the feedback provided from your own body.

In this regard, you might consider the RCP to be like a recipe book. When people first begin to learn how to cook, they typically follow the recipe instructions by rote, without experimentation. It takes time for them to improve their cooking skills, learning how to make the meals they prepare even more flavorful and delicious. But with time, and by heeding their own taste buds and their body's physiological responses to the meals they eat, they soon begin to discover what produces the best results for them in the kitchen. Then, with a bit more experience and confidence under their proverbial belt, they progress further and make the recipes their own.

I encourage you to take the same approach with the RCP, keeping in mind that it is not a fixed solution to health, and never was intended to be. It continues to evolve and to be updated as my scientific explorations continue and also take into account the feedback from practitioners and lay people alike who are now following and using the RCP. My hope is that one day soon, you too will also be providing me similar feedback. For now, read the forthcoming chapters with an open mind, then put what you learn from them into your own daily practice.

We've already covered a lot of ground so far in this book, and there is more awaiting you in the remaining chapters. As you read on, please take enough time so that you fully internalize the RCP's principles and the corresponding information.

I want to emphasize that one of the biggest challenges that people face as they learn these principles and information is letting go of their long-held and deep-seated beliefs about disease and medicine. What this book is intended to do is to peel back the onion layers of these beliefs so that you realize the valid and well-documented scientific information that exists that challenges rather thoroughly the mainstream medicine worldview. Their greatest challenge for practitioners today is that they have come to confuse their "training" with the "truth." No, they are NOT the same.

Essentially, as you move from the science that you learned about in the previous chapters to the practical applications of the RCP that Part Two instructs you in, you are going to unplug yourself from the "medical matrix" that has failed to provide you with more energy and better health, and has only provided you with superficial symptom care. You are about to take that "red pill" so that you can experience firsthand the value that the RCP has for each one of us.

Test everything out for yourself, heeding the wisdom of your body at all times. As you become more familiar with each of the STOPS and STARTS of the RCP, by all means continue to experiment and fine-tune them to suit your individual needs. Just as important, have fun with putting what you learn to use. Never feel that you have to follow the RCP to the letter. Create the best version of it for yourself, so that you will want to, indeed love to, follow it.

PART

Do-It-Yourself Action Steps
To Create Greater Energy and
Better Health

6

Stress, Fatigue, and the Root Cause Protocol

"Stress is the body's inability to make energy for the mind to respond to its environment."

– Mark Hyman, MD

"It's not the stress that kills us, it's our reaction to it..."
– Hans Selye, MD, PhD, ScD, considered the
"Father of Stress Research"

In this chapter, we are going to take a deeper look at stress and how it sets the stage for persistent fatigue. Then, I will provide you with an overview of the Root Cause Protocol itself and explain the tests I recommend to best determine your current health status, including how you can obtain them, and what their optimal values should be. But before exploring and explaining the Stress <> Fatigue dynamic, it's important that we understand the basics of mineral life on this planet.

Stress–Our Ever-Present Scourge

In order to understand the full impact of "stress" on our lives, let's start with some key facts that will help to frame why this topic is so important, especially given our unique stance within the Root Cause Protocol on the central relationship between stress, low energy, and many health symptoms. Here are some compelling facts that make life on Planet Earth so unique:

- Iron, at ~35 percent, is the #1 element
- Iron is considered by iron biologists and toxicologists to be the master pro-oxidant element
- Oxygen, despite its prevalence today, was not always on this planet, and did not appear in significant amounts in our atmosphere until ~2.05 - 2.4 billion years ago, in what astrobiologists call the G.O.E., aka the "Great Oxidation Event." The significance of this event is that when there was only 0.1% of oxygen in the air, that small amount of gas eliminated 99 percent of life on the planet. Anaerobic life dominated the planet at that time. Then, with oxygen's appearance, it disappeared!
- Today, there is 21 percent (technically, 20.8 percent for you purists out there) oxygen in the air and this gas is considered to be the second most reactive element on the planet, after fluorine.
- When iron mixes with oxygen, outside our body, it is called "rust." When iron mixes with oxygen, inside our body, it is called "oxidative stress," which is nothing more than a fancy term for rust. The oxygen bound to that iron becomes unusable, which is a key concept for our counter-cultural premise.

These are important facts about our environment that you may or may not have heard before. Now here's the part that I'm quite confident you've never heard:

Bioavailable copper is the sole element on the planet that enabled aerobic life to form long ago, and it is what enables all animals to harness the "energy" that the oxygen molecule represents, and naturally complexed copper does so without creating any "exhaust."

To recap what you learned in Part One of this book, copper activates oxygen (O2) to enable energy production in our mitochondria, and deactivates oxidants (accidents with oxygen) to ensure exhaust gets eliminated from our mitochondria and cells. In addition, copper incorporates oxygen into a series of key enzymes to regulate metabolic transactions in our body.

The G.O.E. noted above was met with the simultaneous appearance of several important copper metabolites according to the fossil records dating from that historic time. These include:

- KEY copper enzymes, called "multi-copper oxidases" that turn O2 into 2H2O.
- Melatonin, a powerful antioxidant enzyme found inside our mitochondria, that does much more than ensure our sleep.
- And cholesterol. To produce one molecule of cholesterol requires 11 molecules of oxygen. Isn't it intriguing that cholesterol, one of the oldest elements on the planet, has a profound historical relationship with copper, yet is treated as a "disease" by practitioners that do not understand mineral metabolism, oxygen metabolism, nor energy metabolism? More about that in later chapters.

Despite the chest-beating to the contrary, bioavailable copper is essential for proper regulation of methylation functions throughout the body (Jaiser and Winston, 2010), and furthermore, the lack of bioavailable copper has a decided impact on our gene expression. It is noteworthy that scientists know that copper deficiency increases oxidative stress (rust) in our body. Leslie M. Klevay, MD, ScD, in a series of key studies (1973; 1975; 1977 & 1978) demonstrated that copper deficiency causes the rise of oxidative stress that is naturally met with an increase in cholesterol production in our body. Said another way, high cholesterol is a clinical sign of high oxidative stress that is a clinical sign of low bioavailable copper. These are an important series of connection for fully understanding the role that copper, stress and oxidative stress play in our symptoms, our blood tests, and our prescriptions.

Stress is a ubiquitous part of life. So much so that many people underestimate how much stress affects them on an ongoing basis. According to researchers such as Bruce Lipton, PhD, stress is the single most important cause of more than 95 percent of all diseases. (I would assert that it's likely closer to 100 percent.) This should hardly be surprising.

When we talk about stress in our lives, it is important that we understand that this stress outside our body, becomes oxidative stress inside our cells. This is one of the most overlooked dimensions of life on this planet. As soon as copper becomes compromised in our body, it is axiomatic that we will then be dealing with metabolic, oxidative stress, given copper's unique and central role on the planet: harness oxygen to *create energy* and to *clear exhaust*. I find it fascinating that no doctor school—that I know of—distills the essence of metabolism down to these primal and critical mineral and metabolic facts.

Making matters worse, every time you experience stress, your body's supply of magnesium, the foremost anti-stress mineral and nutrient, is rapidly diminished. More about how and why this magnesium dimension is so important in just a moment.

The factors that trigger stress are many, varied and ubiquitous because they are found in all areas of our lives, occurring within four major categories—physical, emotional, environmental, and metabolic. This model is based on the pioneering work of Mildred S. Seelig, MD, MPH (1980), who showed that a relentless loss of magnesium follows each of these four categories of stress. Based upon her amazing body of research, I coined the phrase, Magnesium Burn Rate, or MBR. While there are many stress factors falling into those four categories noted above, there is but one stress response, which was shown by Carl Ludwig Alfred Fiedler, MD, a famed Viennese physician who developed his model of stress response in 1899:

- Stress causes magnesium loss
- Magnesium loss causes electrolyte loss
- Electrolyte loss causes energy loss
- Energy loss causes cell death
- Cell death triggers the natural bodily response of inflammation to clear dead tissue
- Inflammation is followed by the natural bodily response of calcification and fibrosis.

I now understand that one of the key stressors that he is referring to—oxidative stress—is triggered by too little copper that causes too much iron to then accumulate in the tissue. That excess, unbound iron then causes increased oxidative stress and a loss of magnesium, and that loss then invites increased calcification. Know that the connections between iron dysregulation and calcification are many and varied in the scientific research that addresses and examines mineral metabolism.

Again, this stress response is triggered regardless of the originating source or origin of stress.

When stress originating outside our body is pronounced or acute we know it. We've all felt that agonizing sensation in our gut when such stressors hit us. But oftentimes we may not be aware of the hidden stressors, the "metabolic" stressors, particularly stress caused by poor diet, nutrient imbalances or deficiencies, as well as exposures to EMFs and environmental toxins. Given that we live on a planet with 21 percent "pO2ison" (oxygen) in the air, and therefore in our body, and that only one element, copper, can "harness" this oxygen, a lack of bioavailable copper would cause significant "oxidative" (think, "metabolic") stress in our cellular pathways, tissues, organs, and throughout our body. Therefore, lack of bioavailable copper stands to be among the greatest forms of stress that we can experience while residing on this planet. It's an intriguing thought that belies the oft-expressed, but little understood phrase of "copper toxicity!"

It's likely that you've never considered low bioavailable copper as a cause for your ailments. Which begs the obvious question: Are there any research studies that suggest that low bioavailable copper is a dietary, metabolic or environmental stress factor? Yes, indeed, there are. In fact, there are literally thousands of such studies, but your doctor is not aware of any of them, and neither are you. Why? As we discussed previously, minerals are not in the wheelhouse of conventional and many alternative practitioners. Minerals do not generate notable income. That said, here are four noteworthy studies to frame this discussion:

- Cartwright & Wintrobe, 1964, "The Question of Copper Deficiency in Man"
- Picco, Dulout et al, 2004, "Association Between Copper Deficiency and DNA Damage in Cattle" (Please don't be

fooled by the "cattle," there are MANY mentions of humans in this study!)

- Zentek and Meyer, 1991, "Investigations on Copper Deficiency in Growing Dogs"
- Klevay, 1990, "The Effects of Dietary Copper Deficiency and Psychological Stress on Blood Pressure in Rats"

Each of these studies, as well as hundreds of others that I could have selected, explore the profound impact that low bioavailable copper has on energy production, metabolic functions, DNA metabolism, and proliferation of symptoms in the experimental groups, whether they be 2-legged or 4-legged creatures. Despite the wide divergence of animals being studied, the impacts are similar, strikingly similar! It turns out that all life on this planet, and especially the animals must have bioavailable copper to manage and "harness" the oxygen found on this planet.

Each of these studies also offers important findings about the impact that low bioavailable copper has on our inability to respond to metabolizing oxygen and thereby potentially generate oxidative stress. This is a very important point. There is a specific reason why I'm emphasizing this, particularly at this time on the planet.

Whether you are aware of stress or not, does not matter. In either case, once stress occurs— it makes no difference whether it is in response to something real or is due to a conscious or unconscious reaction to a "paper tiger" based on our (mis)perceptions; the stress response is the same—our bodies experience a surge of stress hormones, especially cortisol, the grand-daddy of the adrenal glands, to ensure that we have enough energy to mobilize a response to the crisis. Under the right conditions, this "fight or flight" syndrome response is supposed to subside once the danger (stress trigger), real or not, is over. At least, that was the case for most of human existence.

Even animals experience this same dynamic, but it seems that they are far better at recovering from stress than we modern-day humans are. As Robert M. Sapolsky, PhD explained in his wonderful book *Why Zebras Don't Get Ulcers*, what's notable is that animals in the wild are constantly faced with stress— it's an absolute in nature. Yet, animals don't experience the same chronic symptoms that we humans do as a result of stress. After being chased by a lion, once they escape, they are able to effortlessly calm down and take a relaxing drink.

Now why is that?

I set out to get a better handle on that, because it didn't make sense to me. What I found lurking in the shadows were our friends and faithful companions, magnesium and copper—or their lack thereof. It turns out that there are two key stress hormones in our bodies. One of them, cortisone, is the inactive form, and the other, cortisol, is the active form. Do you know when your body is releasing these stress hormones?

No! Like using up the gasoline in your car, it's a slow and steady drain. These stress hormones cause the loss of cellular magnesium leading directly to problems with cellular energy production, and skeletal and heart muscle performance that lead to blood clotting and heart arrhythmias. But in a body (both human or animal) that has plenty of copper and magnesium, there is a natural process of acting on the impulse of these very strong hormones, and then being able to "calm down," naturally and effortlessly.

But humans in modern times, especially in the past few decades, seem to have lost this natural ability to react to and then recover from stress properly, the way that animals in the wild do, and the way our ancestors before us did. What happened in modern times to cause this change that has increasingly turned growing numbers of humans into "stress victims?"

Well, for one thing, as you learned in Chapter 2, we've created a stark and unhealthy deficiency of copper, as well as magnesium, in our crop soil and food supply, leaving nearly everyone perpetually copper and magnesium deficient. As anybody who's followed my recommendations over the years knows, I'm quick to tell folks who are overwhelmed with stress to *"Take Mo' Maggie!"* With good reason. We are learning with increasing frequency that magnesium is nature's very own "chill pill," as *Psychology Today* noted years ago. (www.psychologytoday.com/blog/evolutionary-psychiatry/201106/ magnesium-and-the-brain-the-original-chill-pill)

As Emily Deans, MD, the author of that article stated, "Our ancestors would have had a ready supply [of magnesium] from organ meats, seafood, mineral water, and even swimming in the ocean, but modern soil can be depleted of minerals and magnesium is removed from water during routine municipal treatment...[and] stress causes use to waste our magnesium like crazy."

It is magnesium that provides us with "calm energy." And there's actually an inverse relationship between cortisol and magnesium. When our bodies' magnesium stores are down, or depleted—and they would be when we are under stress—cortisol levels spike upward. In addition, stress makes our bodies more acidic. Magnesium is used to buffer that acid and stress causes you to burn magnesium faster to neutralize that rise in acid.

Moreover, as stress depletes you of magnesium, low intracellular magnesium causes the excretion of MORE stress hormones. The stress hormones also signal the body to release free fatty acids as an energy source. However, there is a price to pay for this extra needed energy boost during times of stress. These free fatty acids bind and inactivate magnesium in you blood stream and heart, slowing down the transport of glucose and oxygen into muscles and preventing magnesium from being used to make ATP as energy, using a more inefficient free fatty acid source for energy. Fatigue, cellular oxygen deprivation especially of heart tissue, increased free radicals, loss of glucose transport, and our cholesterol ratios are thrown out of balance. The end result is that we hit a wall energetically.

But that's far from the entire story. Other key players that determine how well or poorly our bodies manage stress are enzymes known as the 11beta-hydroxysteroids (11B-HSD1 & 11B-HSD2), which manage the conversion of cortisone into cortisol and back.

And back, you say?

Yes. You see, our body is supposed to effortlessly move back and forth between *"fight and flight"* (sympathetic state) and *"rest and recovery"* (parasympathetic state). Here's the biological equation that runs this pathway for those readers who are interested in the actual biochemistry involved (please forgive my geekiness):

11Beta-Hydroxysteroid + NADP+ ⟺ 11Beta-Oxysteroid + NADPH + H+

(NADP+ stands for nicotinamide adenine dinucleotide phosphate; NADPH is the reduced, or redox, form of NADP+, and H+ stand for a hydrogen ion.) What the above equation shows is that it is this enzyme, 11beta-Hydroxysteroid Dehydrogenase type 2 (11-BHDT2), that converts cortisone into cortisol to deal with stress, and then back to cortisone once the stress crisis is over.

But what does that have to do with magnesium, you may ask?

Good question, and, initially, I wasn't certain, so I kept digging through the scientific literature. Then I came across this article: [www. biochemj.org/bj/338/0229/3380229.pdf]. It clearly explains that the very mechanism to convert NADP+ into NADPH requires magnesium.

Without sufficient magnesium, the conversion of NADP+ into NADPH cannot occur. Which, in turn, means that there can be no recycling of cortisol back to its storage state, so that it doesn't become toxic to our bodies. This is but one of the literally thousands of roles that magnesium plays in our bodies — non-stop, day-in and day-out. Which is why I stand by my recommendation: *When your feel your body's stress response accelerating, take Mo' Maggie* (more magnesium). That's a basic tenet of the Root Cause Protocol.

There is even more to this story, and it has to do with...can you guess it? That's right—iron!

This was made clear in a fascinating and important study published in the *Journal of Bacteriology* in October 2009 (Sandrini SM, et al.), which conclusively showed that stress hormones cause iron to be liberated from lactoferrin and transferrin, both of which serve as vital immune defense proteins. Prior to this study, it was a well-known fact (apparently not embraced by doctors and medical schools, however!) that stress hormones "stimulate the growth of infectious bacteria." In addition, as the researchers of this study point out, "Iron is a key nutritional element required for the growth of almost all bacteria." (Ibid)

Let's connect the dots to understand the importance of what this study has established:

1. Iron is necessary for the growth of virtually all bacteria in your body.
2. Stress hormones release iron to make it more widely available to bacteria.
3. This, in turn, makes it easier for bacteria to proliferate (grow) in your body.
4. Unchecked bacterial growth in your body causes your body's defense and energy-producing mechanisms to be diverted away from other bodily processes in order to cope with the bacteria.
5. As a result, your body lacks the energy it needs to perform its other functions, setting the stage for fatigue and, eventually, disease.

No wonder stress is said to be responsible for 95 percent of all illness!

The findings of this study also further explain why magnesium is the first mineral to be depleted by stress. This happens as a reaction to the mobilized iron that is freed by stress hormones so that bacteria can latch on to it.

Guess what turns off these stress hormones?

Ceruloplasmin! Specifically, because of how an enzyme known as amine oxidase acts through ceruloplasmin to shut down the actions of these stress hormones. That is one of the 24 known functions of ceruloplasmin, our body's master antioxidant stress protein.

Now that we understand these basic relationships and functions, let me add an additional layer to this dynamic. It involves the impact that cortisol has on copper. It is a major issue that is not widely understood in conventional, nor alternative practitioner circles. The release of cortisol, whether from the action of ACTH (responding to magnesium deficiency) or the increased expression of cytokine IL-1B (responding to rising levels of iron), triggers the four-fivefold increase in metallothionein (MT) protein. Why is this a problem? MT has known properties to bind up copper one thousand times stronger than it binds up zinc. (Picture someone who is twice as strong as you—maybe three times as strong—we can't even imagine what 1,000 times stronger means!) This MT action takes bioavailable copper out of action. This then lowers our energy production and that then weakens our immune system function and intelligence. These are all the known downstream effects of chronic stress, and chronic cortisol release. What we are now understanding are the key mineral and metabolic dynamics that are driving these predictable biological stress reactions.

Clearly, the management of these three key minerals is paramount: magnesium, copper, and iron. Their impact on this key enzyme to regulate cortisol release or return it to storage is a critical piece of the puzzle that is known to few who treat "chronic fatigue." Now, here's where it gets interesting.

Copper deficiency >> INC Hyperlipidemic Mice >> INC Exp of 11B-HSD-1. (INC = Increase; 11B-HSD-1 = 11Beta-Hydroxysteroid Dehydrogenase-1)

This relationship is a very significant dynamic. Despite what most might think, most people are copper deficient. Thus, when faced with chronic stressors, we, too, have the potential to respond just like "hyperlipidemic mice" and keep cortisol in its active state via 11B-HSD-1. But when this critical enzyme is silenced, it stops atherosclerosis, the number one cause of death on the planet. What the research clearly shows is that increased 11B-HSD-1 results in the following metabolic events:

- Increased aortic cholesterol
- Increased total cholesterol
- Increased triglycerides
- Increased accumulation of oxidized ("rusted") lipids
- Decreased expression of Nrf2 (This is the genetic key to antioxidant enzymes which are designed to stop oxidative stress.)
- Increased hypertension

So, we have compelling and powerful proof of the impact that stress has on our mineral status and subsequently on our metabolic status. So why is it important to understand all of this, especially as the world community struggles to respond to SARS-CoV-2? Well, you might have noted that I listed a key study (1990) on the impact of restraint on copper-deficient rats by Leslie M. Klevay, MD, ScD. The impact of restraint has an undeniable negative impact on our health and well-being.

Now here's the punch line: Noted below are two key studies that present a 1-2 punch to this material:

- Zaminpira et al, 2019-Dec, "How Chronic Fear Results In Hypoxia in Tissues andCancer in Humans through Bohr Effect"

- Chen et al, 2020-Sep, "Restraint Stress Alters Expression of Glucocorticoid [Cortisol] Bioavailability Mediators, Suppresses Nrf2, and Promotes Oxidative Stress in Liver Tissue"

What these two studies do is present a powerful argument that the emotion of fear triggers the metabolic state of hypoxia (the first stage of oxidative stress), and this triggers the release of both cortisol and adrenaline. The meticulous connections that Zaminpira et al (2019) make are stunning. Then, syncing that information up with the Chen et al (2020) study we see the full-scale impact of restraint via an *in vivo* study of humans. The conclusion of this latter study says it all: *"Stress-induced oxidative stress appears to generate a tissue-specific response that in the liver is characterized by a robust and antithetical reduction in the Nrf2-Keap1-ARE signaling pathway. This results in substantial reductions in GSH/cysteine thiol-mediated cellular antioxidant capacity and increased oxidative damage to lipids and proteins. Moreover, despite high levels of circulating glucocorticoids, local hepatic tissue levels of corticosterone are likely potentiated further by a systematic increase in bioavailability mediated by reduced protein binding and increased reactivation."* Clearly, we need to get a handle on our stressors and learn to regulate our mineral intake via our diet and the nutrients highlighted in the RCP.

Understanding all of the above does not require a degree in rocket science.

Moreover, these concepts are clearly proven to be borne out repeatedly in the medical literature. Sadly, though, this is not something doctors have been taught. Minerals, especially magnesium and copper, are not part of the medical curricula, and the mention of ceruloplasmin (Cp)in medical schools is, for all intents and purposes, akin to mentioning "Voldemort" at Hogwarts Academy. It appears that ceruloplasmin is the master antioxidant stress protein *"that which must **not** be named."*

Fortunately, you don't need to go to medical school, nor do you need to rely on doctors who have never been taught these concepts, in order to protect yourself from the ravages of stress and its resultant fatigue and illness. You can gain all the protection you need on your own by following the Root Cause Protocol. By doing so, you will continually be supplying your body with the magnesium, copper, and ceruloplasmin it needs, while keeping iron in proper metabolic check, to join the thousands of others who have gained more energy and greater resilience to stress because of how the RCP has helped them.

Finally, what we place priority emphasis on in our health consultations via the RCPCs (Root Cause Protocol Consultants) is starting with understanding the clients' "Story of Stress" throughout their lifetime, and especially in the time period just prior to the onset of key symptoms. We want to know when the symptoms began, and then delve into what dimensions of stress were dominating our clients' lives prior to the onset of those symptoms. Now that we have a detailed understanding of how stress causes mineral dysregulation, this approach makes perfect sense. The testing that we routinely employ is used as a tool to prove, via the results in the mineral assessments, HTMA and blood test, just how much their minerals were affected by the experienced pattern(s) of stress. It is a powerful moment when the client realizes that their stress, and *not* some "medical disease" was the *true* origin of their symptoms and their medical label. We have found this to be a very enlightening and empowering dynamic that galvanizes clients into action and further adoption of the principles and practices of the RCP (Root Cause Protocol). Given that, let's now turn our attention to better understanding the tenets and facets of the RCP.

An Overview of The Root Cause Protocol

As you learned in Part One of this book, the aim of the Root Cause Protocol is to increase bioavailable copper in order to decrease the accumulation of unbound iron in your body, while simultaneously reducing what I call your body's magnesium burn rate (MBR), meaning the rate in which your body's supply of magnesium is depleted, or "burned up." By accomplishing this, the RCP repairs the mineral imbalances that are the root cause of both persistent fatigue and nearly all other health challenges you may face.

Stated more scientifically, the RCP is designed to help the body "make" the copper-dependent protein, ceruloplasmin and "empower" its ferroxidase enzyme activity, in order to reduce oxidative stress and inflammation. Ceruloplasmin, in a healthy body, among many enzyme functions, enables ferroxidase function. Ferroxidase (FOX), the "active" form of ceruloplasmin, is the enzyme that regulates, or "chaperones," iron and prevents it from allowing oxidation ("rusting") to occur. Ferroxidase is the master antioxidant enzyme that regulates iron status in the body. Dysregulated, unbound iron is the greatest source of oxidative stress and inflammation in the body. Remember:

> Bioavailable copper converts toxic ferrous iron (Fe ++) into beneficial ferric iron (Fe +++).

> Without enough bioavailable copper, unbound toxic ferrous iron runs around the body like a four-year-old with a hammer, causing oxidative stress and inflammation which are the root cause of virtually all health challenges.

> Therefore, the priority focus of the Root Cause Protocol is to increase bioavailable copper, which will minimize oxidative stress and ultimately, minimize the magnesium burn rate (MBR).

Let's briefly recap the roles that each of these elements play in our body so that we can better understand these concepts. Ultimately, we want to ensure that they work the way nature intended, thereby keeping us healthy and full of energy.

Copper: Copper is responsible for many profound functions in the body, and is principally focused on creating energy via cytochrome c oxidase, and clearing exhaust within a network of antioxidant enzymes, in what I call the body's Integrated Antioxidant System. But in order for copper to be able to perform its functions, it must be bioavailable, meaning that it needs to be "complexed" in a network of proteins and enzymes. This doesn't happen magically. Ninety-five percent of copper in the blood is "complexed" in ceruloplasmin. However, for copper to be loaded in ceruloplasmin, we need the critical involvement of retinol, which is an essential nutrient for this process. Following the Root Cause Protocol ensures that you obtain enough retinol to do its job. *This is important, because taking dietary copper supplements will not increase the amount of bioavailable copper inside your body.*

Ceruloplasmin: Ceruloplasmin was discovered in the early 1940s by the Swedish physiologists Carl G.Holmberg and C.B. Laurell, and first described in their article published in 1948. Since its discovery, ceruloplasmin has been revealed to be the master "multi-copper protein." It has an "active" and an "inactive" state, or is measured via its "enzyme activity" or its level of "immunoreactive protein." In its "active" state, ceruloplasmin contains up to eight copper atoms, several of which surround a molecule of oxygen (O_2). But unfortunately, only the level of the "inactive" state is measured by commercial labs using the serum ceruloplasmin blood test. Outside of research studies, there are no commercial labs that measure the "active" state. The Root Cause Protocol, however, helps to ensure that ceruloplasmin actively and properly complexes the needed copper for its many enzyme and regulatory actions.

Ferroxidase (FOX): Ferroxidase is one of the key "active," or "enzyme" forms of ceruloplasmin. FOX is the master antioxidant enzyme in the human body. Most importantly, it regulates iron and prevents it from causing oxidative stress, aka "rust," in the body's tissues and organs. Ferroxidase has the highest amount of activity in the liver and the brain, and is also notably active in our intestines, where it is expressed through a protein called hephaestin, and, in pregnant women, in the placenta, this enzyme is expressed through the protein zyklopen. (It is worth noting that pregnant women express three forms of bioavailable copper, and yet contemporary obstetrics and midwifery do not test for copper status, nor any of these enzymes. The management of iron and oxygen is critical to the developing fetus, as you might expect.)

Without optimal ferroxidase enzyme activity, iron starts to build up in our tissues, especially in our liver cells and endocrine (hormone) glands. As we age, this chronic build-up of iron leads to decreased energy production in the cells, and increased inflammation in our tissues and organs.

Increasing the amount of ceruloplasmin in the body and the activity of the ferroxidase enzyme is *the priority focus* of the recommended steps in The Root Cause Protocol. *By increasing ceruloplasmin and ferroxidase action, we decrease iron dysfunction, we increase the potential to activate oxygen for energy production, and we stop the chronic loss of magnesium.*

Magnesium: This key mineral as we noted previously is responsible for 3,751 essential enzyme functions in the body. Among its many functions, magnesium regulates calcium homeostasis through the activity of three key hormones: calcitonin, parathyroid hormone, and vitamin D (more properly called "hormone D"). In addition, magnesium's presence in the energy molecule (Mg-ATP) is an absolute requirement for its recognition and use in the body. I consider magnesium to be the "conductor of the body's mineral orchestra."

Magnesium Burn Rate (MBR): Under any form of stress to the body (physical, emotional, metabolic, environmental, etc.), magnesium is lost as a metabolic response, because when the body is under stress, it needs to produce more energy, (Mg-ATP), which requires it to call upon its magnesium stores. Under extreme and/or sustained stress—and a failure to properly re-mineralize—the body loses its natural ability to respond to stress, causing oxidative stress and inflammation to build up throughout the body. Magnesium deficiency, meaning low magnesium levels in red blood cells, where magnesium belongs, is the recognized precursor to inflammation.

However, when the body is expressing optimal ferroxidase activity, the MBR will be at a minimum. The Root Cause Protocol is designed to help ensure this.

Retinol: Retinol is the naturally occurring, animal-based, whole-food form of fat soluble vitamin A. It is found in cod liver oil, beef liver, butter from grass-fed cows, and other animal-based foods. Retinol is vital for "loading" copper into ceruloplasmin, so that it can then regulate iron as needed throughout the body, while preventing it from causing inflammation and oxidative stress.

Once I began to understand how important all of the above nutrients are to our health and energy levels, I set out on a mission to find the best solution that anyone could use to achieve the restoration and maintenance of the proper balance of the above nutrients and enzymes. That is how I came to develop the Root Cause Protocol. It began with one STOP and one START, and has since evolved over the years.

I realize many readers may not be interested in fully comprehending the biochemistry involved in the RCP. Most likely, you are one of them, and that's fine. You don't have to fully understand it for the RCP to work for you, any more than you have to truly know how electricity works to get the benefit of turning on a light switch in the dark. Though the biochemistry involved in the RCP may seem complex to you, putting it to use is actually quite simple, though it does require a commitment on your part if you want it to truly work for you.

There are really only two steps you need to follow, which I have divided into two categories called the STOPS and the STARTS. In the next chapter, you will learn much more about each of these categories and what they involve. For now, let me just say that if I had to state the *most important* thing that you need to achieve in order to vanquish fatigue and have more energy and improved health, it would be *increasing ferroxidase function* in your body.

I've spent many years researching the peer-reviewed, scientific literature from around the world (dating back to 1948) on the subject of how to increase ferroxidase function. This body of research clearly shows that each of the STOPS of the Root Cause Protocol disrupt, or STOP, the proper ferroxidase function. And, conversely, each of the STARTS in the RCP improve ferroxidase function.

Here is a list of the 12 most important items I recommend you stop doing immediately:

1) **STOP** taking iron supplements
2) **STOP** taking vitamin D3 supplements
3) **STOP** taking calcium supplements
4) **STOP** taking zinc supplements
5) **STOP** taking molybdenum supplements
6) **STOP** taking "drugstore" once-a-day multivitamins, prenatal vitamins, etc.
7) **STOP** Taking B Vitamins from a bottle (get them from food)
8) **STOP** using synthetic forms of ascorbic acid (synthetic vitamin C), citrate, and citric acid
9) **STOP** using high fructose corn syrup (HFCS) and synthetic sugars
10) **STOP** using industrialized omega-6 oils (e.g. soybean oil, canola oil, etc.)

11) **STOP** using fluoride (toothpaste, water, etc.)
12) **STOP** using colloidal silver as an antibiotic/antimicrobial (although please know that nano-silver or sovereign silver have different properties and are OK)
13) **STOP** eating low-fat, high-carbohydrate, processed, refined foods
14) **LIMIT** Exposure to environmental toxins, including unchecked blue light exposure

Just stopping these 12 items is likely to make an impact with a notable improvement in your health and energy. (The reasons why are explained in Chapter 7.) Best of all, you can stop all of the above for free, starting right now! So put these STOPS into action and discover for yourself what a positive difference they can make for you.

Determining Your Current State of Health

The best way to reach your destination is to start by knowing where you are. In terms of health, this means starting with an accurate assessment of how healthy you are currently. Doing so and then repeating a follow-up health assessment every six to twelve months can also help you track the progress you are making as you follow the Root Cause Protocol.

To evaluate your health status, I recommend a selection of blood tests, as well as a hair tissue mineral analysis (HTMA), sometimes referred to simply as a hair mineral analysis. Unfortunately, none of these recommended tests are likely to be mentioned by your doctor, nor are they trained in their proper interpretation as it relates to your metabolism.

We are led to believe that the medical system is exhaustive in its blood-testing search for clues to what's right or not right with our health and metabolism. What I have come to discover, however, is that much of the laboratory testing that is commercially available in the United States and around the world is based far more on availability, and not on so much on the tests' clinical accuracy or their applicability to our energy producing processes.

An obvious case in point is that few physicians even consider evaluating their patients' red blood cell magnesium levels, known as the Magnesium RBC test. This is despite magnesium's obvious importance in all 100 trillion cells of our body, as well as some 3,751 proteins, known as the Magnesome. In addition, magnesium is essential to activate 8 of the 10 enzymes for RBCs to make their energy. Instead, practitioners rely on serum (blood) tests that tell us nothing about a person's true magnesium status. Why? Because it is magnesium *inside* the red blood cells that count, not magnesium in the serum, which is the liquid *outside* the red blood cells. The focus of the "spotlight" does make a difference.

Nor do doctors test for ferroxidase enzyme function, the master anti-oxidant enzyme in the human body that no doctor seems to know about. In fact, at present, and quite unfortunately, there are no lab tests available to consumers for measuring ferroxidase function. Given this restriction, it must be "triangulated," based on several blood and hair-tissue markers, as well as overall bodily function and symptoms. This approach is directionally correct, though it is not definitive. As a consultant, I learned long ago that it is far better to do the right things.

These are but two key tests, among other "missing" tests from the typical arsenal that doctors are trained to provide, and allowed to order. Unfortunately, this group of available tests does little to meaningfully pull back the curtain on the true mineral dysregulation that is driving the cellular dynamics of metabolic dysfunction that results in symptoms.

At the end of the day, all we can do is the best that's currently available, but that should not deter us from pointing out the glaring shortages and inadequacies of current laboratory testing for iron status, that drive inconclusive, and at times, faulty clinical conclusions.

Blood Tests: Ultimately, we want to look at the following blood markers:

Serum Iron (Measures the "efficiency" of iron, similar to measuring mile per gallon, or MPG, in a car.)

Total Iron-Binding Capacity (TIBC) and/or Saturation (Measures how many "docking stations" are available for iron.)

Serum Ferritin (Measures the protein that stores iron in the tissues.)

Serum Transferrin (Measures the key "transport" protein that "recycles" iron from tissue back into the bloodstream.)

Serum Copper (Measures the total amount of copper in the blood.)

Serum Ceruloplasmin (Measures the level, NOT the activity, of this marker for bioavailable copper, which regulates iron.)

Red Blood Cell (RBC) Magnesium (Measures the amount of magnesium in the red blood cells.)

Plasma Zinc (Measures the amount of zinc in the plasma/serum.)

Hemoglobin (Measures the amount of this protein responsible for transporting oxygen in the bloodstream.)

Vitamin A (Retinol) (Measures the amount of pre-formed vitamin A in our blood.

Vitamin D (25-OH) (Measures the amount of "storage" vitamin D, or calcidiol, in our blood.)

Vitamin D (1, 25 [OH]2D3 (Measures the amount of "active" vitamin D, or calcitriol, in our blood)

The above tests can be ordered by your doctor, although you may have to explain to him or her why you want them. Fortunately, you do not have to depend on a doctor in order to obtain them, as they are also available from various lab companies that provide blood and other health tests directly to consumers without a doctor's prescription. You will find a listing of such companies in the Resources section.

Note: Different labs in different regions of the world may have different names for any (or all) of the above tests. Please work with the lab and/or your physician if you need to translate them into your local options.

Ideal Values: Everyone wants to know what the "ideal" or "optimal" values should be when they receive their test results. This is a perfectly logical question. But please note that is a very simple question with a very complex answer. Think of it this way: The range of body temperature is 92° – 108°F (or 32° – 45°C). But we know that the "ideal" body temperature is supposed to be 98.6°F (or 37°C). The closer we get to either "bookend," the more likely our symptoms will appear. The closer we get to "ideal," the better. But there will always be variation among individuals, so do not look at lab values in a vacuum apart from your specific, individual symptoms.

That said, the following benchmarks for each test are what we recommend:

> **Serum Iron:** USA: ~100 ug/dL for women, ~120 ug/dL for men; Metric (outside the US): ~17.9 mmol/L for women, ~21.5 mmol/L for men.

> **Total Iron-Binding Capacity (TIBC):** USA: ~285 ug/dL for women, ~340 ug/dL for men; Metric: ~51 ug/dL for women, ~60.9 ug/dL for men. If reported as "% Saturation", should be 25–30%.

> **Serum Ferritin:** USA & Metric: ~20–50 ng/mL.

Serum Transferrin: USA: ~300 mg/dL, or ~3.0 g/L; Metric: ~1.35 mmol/L.

Serum Copper: USA: ~100 ug/dL; Metric: ~15.7 umol/L.

Serum Ceruloplasmin: USA: ~30 mg/dL; Metric: ~0.35 g/L.

Red Blood Cell (RBC) Magnesium: USA: ~6.5 mg/dL; Metric: ~2.67 mmol.

Plasma Zinc: USA: ~100 ug/dL; Metric: ~15.3 umol/L.

Hemoglobin: USA: ~12.5 g/dL for women, ~13.5 g/dL for men; Metric: ~125 g/L for women, ~135 g/L for men.

Vitamin A (Retinol): Your active vitamin A level should be three times higher than your vitamin D level.

Vitamin D (25-OH): USA: ~15–30 ng/mL; Metric: ~37.5–75 nmol/L.

Hair Tissue Mineral Analysis (HTMA)

Although widely ignored, and even disparaged, by most doctors, a hair tissue mineral analysis is an extremely noninvasive and cost-effective screening test you can use to measure the levels of essential minerals in your body, such as calcium, magnesium, and zinc, as well as important mineral ratios. In addition, the HTMA can help determine the amount of harmful heavy metals in your body, especially aluminum, arsenic, beryllium, cadmium, lead, mercury, and uranium.

HTMA has been used as a health screening tool since at least 1965, when the International Atomic Energy Agency began to use it. According to a 1980 report by T.S. Ryabukhin, "Hair was chosen by the I.A.E.A. due to the concentration of minerals in the hair and its reflection of both external and internal contamination." (Ryabukhin, T.S. *International Coordinated Program on Activation*

*Analysis of Trace Element Pollutants in Human Hair."*In Hair, Trace Elements, and Human Illness. Brown, A. C.; Crounse, R. G., ed. Praeger Publications, 1980.)

Our hair contains a representation of all the minerals in our body. HTMA measures this mineral composition to provide indications of what the levels of these minerals, both nutritional, and toxic (heavy metals) are in our tissues. This provides a picture of our body's internal environment and our overall health status. With this information, a properly trained HTMA consultant can interpret the efficiency of your body's many metabolic processes and nutritional status. The HTMA test also helps to reveal our "mineral-stress" pattern. Moreover, unlike blood, urine, and saliva tests, which are only capable of revealing a person's mineral status at the time such tests are performed, HTMA provides an indication of a person's mineral stores over a period of time (at least a few months). Overall, I find it to be a very useful tool for getting at the "root causes" of a person's health issues.

Having a hair tissue mineral analysis done is a very simple procedure. Once you contact a lab that performs HTMA testing (see the Resources section for a list of such labs or an RCPC that can provide this test), you will be sent a collection kit in which to send your hair samples back to the lab.

Proper collection of your hair samples is extremely important. Collected hair samples need to be clean and free of hair dyes or bleach. Permed hair should also not be used. Hair should be collected (cut) from several areas of the back portion of your head, cut as close to your scalp as possible. If your hair is long, cut away excess hair, leaving one to one and a half inches of hair from the root end. (For men who are either bald or who have short hair in a buzz cut, you can use pubic hair samples, although scalp hair is preferable.) The total amount of hair needed is equivalent to about one and one-half tablespoons.

Once your hair samples have been analyzed, the lab will mail or email you a detailed assessment reporting its findings. There are no "optimal" or "ideal" numbers for an HTMA, and results are not correlated to your nutrient intake. These numbers (and their ratios) can be reviewed during consultations with a certified Root Cause Protocol Consultant, or, if the lab, provides them, their own consultants.

Obtaining the above blood tests and an HTMA when you begin to implement the Root Cause Protocol, or soon thereafter, is a good idea. Though doing so is not absolutely essential, knowing your nutritional and mineral status can provide you with a clearer picture of your overall health and serve as a concrete record of where you were when you started the RCP. Follow-up tests as needed can the help verify the progress you are making and pinpoint what, if anything, may be necessary for you to fine tune.

Now let's explore in more detail the STOPS and STARTS of the Root Cause Protocol itself.

That is the topic of Chapter 7.

CHAPTER

7

The STOPS–Challenging Conventional Nutritional Mythology

"If you want a happy ending, that depends, of course, on where you stop your story."

– Orson Welles (1915–1985)

In this chapter I am going to explain more about each of the STOPS of the Root Cause Protocol so that you understand why each of them is so important for you to adopt in order to banish fatigue and get and stay healthier. Again, please keep in mind that the singular and foundational focus of this Protocol is to increase bioavailable copper, the most overlooked and misunderstood element on Earth. It is profoundly important to our objective to enable increased energy production *and* this element and the proteins that carry it are also notably sensitive to numerous nutritional factors that will be examined in this chapter.

As I stated in Chapter 6, I recommend you immediately adopt each of the following measures. Please know that these STOPS are available on printable document from the dedicated book website: **https://cureyourfatiguebook.com/resources** These STOPS are as follows:

STOP Taking Iron Supplements

Having read this far, the reason for not taking iron supplements should now be obvious: Too much dietary and supplemental iron is the single most toxic factor contributing to poor health and fatigue. We are already getting too much iron from our food alone.

To recap what you learned in Chapter 4 about the medical profession's blind spots about iron, there are several reasons why you should never take iron supplements and should also do your best to avoid eating foods to which iron has been added, such as grains and cereals. As we noted previously, please do not confuse "iron dysregulation" with "iron deficiency." They are *not* the same condition.

The first reason for not taking iron supplements is that the justification for taking these supplements is based on blood testing that is misinterpreted or flawed. Doctors and others are in a state of complete confusion about what anemia is, and this is compounded by the fact that medical practitioners have not been trained to interpret iron blood tests correctly and completely.

There are three blood markers to assess iron status: hemoglobin, serum iron, and serum ferritin, The first represents about 75 percent of the body's stores of iron, and is routinely overlooked or misinterpreted. The last, ferritin, I have re-named "*errortin*" for the notoriously incorrect interpretations that have been made on my clients' blood tests. All is not as it seems.

The second, and most important reason is that our physiology was never designed to have supplemental iron. As infants, we are supposed to get an enormous download of iron from our mothers, and are designed to then get 95 percent of our daily iron requirement from a recycling system (RES) that is regulated by bioavailable copper. The other five percent, approximately one mg of iron/day, is supposed to be obtained through our diet, and certainly never through multivitamins and targeted supplements. And most of all, we were never designed to have iron added to our flour and grains via inorganic iron filings, which is literally what is used. These iron filings are the most toxic form of iron you can add. (Jym Moon, PhD, 2008, *Iron: The Most Toxic Metal.* George Ohsawa Macrobiotic Foundation.)

The bottom line is that it's a complete violation of our physiology to be adding supplemental iron. This is metabolic poison to our mitochondria and to the bioavailable copper that they rely upon to make our energy.

STOP Taking Vitamin D3 Supplements

Vitamin D supplements continue to be some of the most recommended supplements (along with synthetic vitamin C, aka ascorbic acid or ascorbate) still being pushed by so-called nutritionally oriented physicians and other "experts." As has been the case since vitamin D supplementation first became popular years ago, however, pro-vitamin D doctors and researchers continue to miss the forest for the trees as they continue to ignore the root cause of diseases in general.

In Chapter 8, I explain the misconceptions about, and dangers of, both vitamin D and synthetic vitamin C/ascorbic acid supplementation in more detail. For now, here are the key facts about vitamin D that you need to know:

The molecule that does all the heavy lifting in your body's immune system is 1,25-dihydroxy vitamin D [1,25(OH)2D3]. This is the bioactive form that is rarely measured. It is not the storage form. The storage form is called 25-hydroxy vitamin D [25(OH)D]. This is the form that is most commonly and routinely measured by lab tests.

So there's a complete misunderstanding in the world of medicine and in society in general when it comes to testing vitamin D levels because the form that is being measured is the blood level of a metabolite that is supposed to be in storage, while the level of the far more important bioactive form is being completely overlooked. It is a scientific fact that all the immune function accolades that storage vitamin D continues to receive are really a result of the work of the *bio-active form* of vitamin D in partnership with the vitamin D receptor (VDR) that must be complexed with RXR, a key nuclear receptor that is a derivative of retinol. (Toell, Polly & Carlberg, 2000-Dec 01, "All natural DR3-type vitamin D response elements show a similar functionality in vitro". *Biochem J.* 352(Pt 2): 301–309.) The immune impact is from the bio-active form of vitamin D. Period.

As noted above, another factor that doctors miss is that in order to have its fullest expression, active vitamin D must be complexed with the nuclear receptor called RXR, which requires retinol, or real vitamin A, which no one takes because all they focus on is vitamin D. So, we have a misunderstanding about what form of vitamin D we need, and a misunderstanding about what our vitamin D levels should be. Furthermore, we are completely unaware of the impact that taking Supplemental D does to our intestinal ability to absorb vitamin A.

In addition, regarding the testing range of the storage form of vitamin D, important research was done in 2013 by Mohammed Amer, MD, and his colleagues at John Hopkins University. They conducted a study of all-cause mortality versus levels of storage D. What they discovered was that there was no clinical benefit to having storage D be above 21 ng/mL (nanograms per milliliter). This is vastly different than the reference range that is used on lab testing which starts at 30 ng/ml and goes up to 100 ng/mL. Anyone who has a normal storage D of 21 ng/mL, according to Dr. Amer, would be told that their level was low based on the standard lab test ranges. That then prompts the practitioner to recommend taking additional vitamin D, either as a drug or as a supplement (vitamin D3). The current lab test ranges were developed by Michael F. Holick, PhD, MD, of Boston University and John J. Cannell, MD at the Vitamin D Council, both of whom are among the biggest promoters of vitamin D supplementation, and who have a well-documented, vested interest in doing so. These tests are based on misleading ranges and the entire focus is on an incorrect form of the vitamin D metabolite.

What is also important to understand is that vitamin D in supplement form (25 dihydroxy vitamin D) is not actually a vitamin at all. It really should be called hormone D, because that's precisely how the it acts in the body, similar to all other hormones. 25 dihydroxy vitamin D is called the storage form for a reason. It's a storage molecule that is supposed to be in storage in our liver. It is not supposed to be in our bloodstream. That's what most doctors completely overlook or fail to fully understand.

Moreover, it's been a known fact since 1962, according to the research of John Ferris, MD, at Yale Medical School, that supplemental vitamin D causes renal (kidney) potassium wasting. That's a very serious condition. Every client I've ever worked with who took supplemental vitamin D had a low potassium reading on their HTMA hair test. It can take years to correct that.

Based on my research, I think probably the most disheartening finding is that taking supplemental vitamin D creates a metabolic demand on the liver to flip it into the bioactive form. This demand uses up magnesium, and the bioactive vitamin D triggers the synthesis of metallothionein, a protein that binds up copper a thousand times stronger than it binds up zinc, as we noted previously. So suddenly we have practitioners chasing a form of vitamin D that's flawed using a range that's flawed, creating potassium wasting, which then leads to a buildup of iron accumulation in the tissue. Then we find out that copper is being bound up by metallothionein and therefore is no longer available for metabolic transactions, and neither is magnesium.

Collectively, this series of events creates a metabolic crisis in our mitochondria.

This is entirely different from what happens when vitamin D is produced in the body when we obtain adequate exposure to sunlight. Most people don't understand the many benefits that come from sunlight. Two of the significant benefits that occur with the sun kissing our skin are that sunlight *activates the breakdown of vitamin A* (aka retinol) into the many retinoids that run our metabolism, and sunlight also *triggers the biosynthesis of vitamin D*. It's important to remember that nothing in nature occurs in isolation. Everything is in relationship, and vitamin A and vitamin D do indeed have a relationship, a very powerful relationship. Contrary to the mind-numbing "D"irections we are given, in my humble opinion, it is ten times more important for sunlight to activate the breakdown of vitamin A into those retinoids our bodies need, than synthesizing vitamin D. Today, all of the optics, all of the programming, and all of the propaganda, if you will, is focused squarely on storage vitamin D. No one talks about retinol, real vitamin A, despite the fact that, back in the 1920s, all of the research was centered around retinol, the first fat-soluble vitamin discovered (Hopkins FG, 1912). Today, that research has, for all intents and purposes, been disregarded and thrown away, despite the Nobel Prize awarded in 1929 to Eijkman and Hopkins for their pioneering work on retinol and vitamins, in general.

STOP Taking Calcium Supplements

While it is certainly true that calcium is essential for optimal health, calcium supplements are not. The truth is that, although they are routinely recommended, especially to women, to prevent or "correct" osteoporosis, calcium carbonate supplements are essentially poison to the body's vital bone-building process, and more importantly, poison to the metabolic processes to make energy. The thinking behind taking calcium supplements is based on testing to measure bone density, especially as we get older, because as we age we are more prone to losing bone mass. While it's true that osteoporosis is about calcium loss (aka the "simple lie"), what is ignored is that bone loss is caused by excess, unbound iron (aka, the "complex truth!"). The research is very clear about iron's negative impact on osteoblast activity (the bone building cells of the body), as well as iron's ability to kill alkaline phosphatase enzyme function and osteoblasts, both of which are essential to make new cellular tissue in the bone matrix.

Central to that process is the need for healthy and plentiful bone marrow. Iron in the bone has a unique way of rusting this bone marrow. In addition, healthy and abundant bone marrow requires lots of retinol which is MIA in the standard diet. Also essential to this process of new bone production are bioavailable copper, magnesium, and about a dozen other key minerals. But copper and magnesium are at the head of the stream because of copper's ability to activate lysyl oxidase, and ascorbate oxidase, as well as magnesium's ability to activate alkaline phosphatase enzyme. These three enzymes are essential for optimal regeneration of the bone matrix.

Among the unique properties of iron is its ability to cause *calcium loss from hard tissue* (the bone), while simultaneously causing *calcium buildup in the soft tissue*, especially our arteries. For this reason, as soon as someone presents with osteoporosis (bone), practitioners should also check for rising indications of atherosclerosis (artery). They are simultaneous events in the body. It turns out that iron activates the enzyme called acid phosphatase, as well as a series of other events that trigger the known process of atherosclerosis, which is triggered by iron-induced oxidative stress. (Manolagas SC et al, 2008, "Defense, Defense, Defense: Scavenging H2O2 While Making Cholesterol." *Endocrinology* 149(7): 3264-3266.)

What doctors fixate on with regard to osteoporosis is the acid phosphatase-induced breakdown of the bone matrix, which releases calcium. Then they seek to try to replace that calcium with calcium supplements. It simply does *not* work that way in our body.

In order to replace calcium, you need to be able to activate another equally important enzyme, alkaline phosphatase, which is a critical bone building enzyme which requires magnesium to activate it. When alkaline phosphatase is in play, it is able to replace and restore the lost calcium as part of the bone matrix. The problem with most supplements is that they have a ratio of two parts calcium to one part magnesium, which *blocks* magnesium absorption. Yet, in 2013, QiDai, MD, PhD, a research scientist at Vanderbilt University, proved that when you take two parts magnesium to one part calcium, this ratio *guarantees* calcium absorption. (Dai Q et al, 2013, "Modifying Effect of Calcium/Magnesium Intake Ratio and Mortality: A Population-based Cohort Study." *BMJ Open* 3(2):e002111.)

For years, doctors and nutritionists alike have emphasized calcium at the expense of magnesium, recommending that calcium intake be twice that of magnesium (a 2:1 ratio). Now we know better. The ideal ratio between calcium and magnesium should be 1:1, just as it is in most vegetables, seeds and nuts, the food groups that are rich in both minerals.

Additionally, unlike magnesium, we can obtain all of our calcium needs solely through our diet. What throws our metabolism off is the addition of calcium supplements. This sends the body's calcium stores out of balance, leading to excessive levels that prevent the proper uptake and utilization of magnesium. Therefore, it's not surprising—at least not to me—that calcium supplementation is now being shown by research to cause calcification in the body, including in the arteries. (Reid and Bolland, 2010; 2011; 2012; 2013; 2014; 2015; 2016.)

Keep in mind, during all the years of human existence on this planet, prior to the 20th century, our diet contained an ideal 1:1 balance of calcium to magnesium. But starting about 100 years ago, our food started to change, in large part due to refining, the advent of commercial farming, the introduction of thousands of food additives, and the prevalence of carbohydrate-rich grains and carbonated drinks. As a result, as only America could, we have now created a dietary Ca/Mg ratio of almost 5:1, nearly a 500 percent increase from where it needs to be. (Rosanoff A, et al, 2012-Feb 15, "Suboptimal Magnesium Status in the United States: Are the Health Consequences Underestimated?" *Nutritional Reviews* 70(3).)

Not only that, but dairy products, which were a limited part of our ancient ancestors' far healthier diet, and yet are now the most commonly recommended calcium-rich foods, also have an unhealthy Ca/Mg ratio. Pasteurized, homogenized milk, for instance, contains seven parts calcium to one part magnesium, while commercial yogurts and cheeses are even worse (11:1 and 26:1, respectively). These dairy products also contain the synthetic form of vitamin D (D2), which, as you learned above, further damages our mineral balances, and ultimately our health.

STOP Taking Zinc Supplements

Zinc is another nutrient that you should only obtain through your diet, not as a supplement. Since at least 2010, research by James A. Duce, PhD at the University of Melbourne and others have proven that zinc kills the ferroxidase enzyme function of B-amyloid protein precursor. (Duce et al, 2010, "An Iron-Export Ferroxidase Activity of B-Amyloid Protein Precursor is Inhibited by Zinc in Alzheimer's Disease" *Cell* 142(6): 857-867.) As you learned earlier in this book, ferroxidase is responsible for the conversion of reactive, oxidative ferrous iron (Fe++) into the bound form of ferric iron (Fe3+) found in transferrin and ferritin, which prevents Fe2+ from causing oxidative stress (free radical damage) by generating superoxide, hydrogen peroxide, and the most destructive biomolecules of all, the hydroxyl radicals.

Beyond that, zinc supplements, unlike dietary zinc, trigger the production of metallothionein in the liver. Again, please keep in mind that metallothionein binds up copper a thousand times greater than it binds up zinc. The significance of that function is that what you've done is effectively taken the source of copper, which is the liver, out of the system, and thereby out of the metabolic process to make energy. As you've also learned, one of the mechanisms of ceruloplasmin is that it's a copper transport protein, acting like a supply line for the mitochondria within the body. There is a rich legacy of world-renowned research from the 1960s to 2017 that documents and demonstrates this critical copper transport function. As an analogy, picture an army, An army travels on its stomach. If it doesn't have the supplies it needs, it can't move and can't perform. Similarly, if ceruloplasmin can't transport copper, the mitochondria can't produce all of the energy our body needs, resulting in fatigue– notably symptoms and ultimately, metabolic dysfunction.

Zinc was not considered to have much importance as far as energy production and immune function until the 1960s. Prior to that, luminary scientists such as Otto H. Warburg, PhD, MD, Heinrich O. Weiland. PhD, and others, in their hunt to discover what creates energy in the body, were focusing on copper and iron. Zinc didn't enter the clinical and nutritional scene until the 1960s, beginning with the work of Carl C Pfeiffer, MD, PhD, at Princeton University, who claimed that there is a ratio between copper and zinc that is important and which must be kept in balance.

Pfeiffer's work influenced William Walsh, PhD, an electrical engineer, who brought attention to compounds called kryptopyrroles, which can occur as byproducts of hemoglobin synthesis (hemoglobin is the molecule that carries oxygen in our blood). Walsh and others recognized that when kryptopyrroles are present, they can cause a loss of zinc and vitamin B6. They then mistakenly concluded that to correct the presence of kryptopyrroles we need to flood the body with zinc and B6. In reality, that's the worst thing you can do. You correct kryptopyrroles by correcting the process of making new blood cells with bioavailable copper. This dependence on copper to make new blood has been known and studied extensively since the 1920s, yet it is simply *not* taught in any doctor school.

What Walsh and others failed to understand is that the last step in the production of heme (the oxygen-carrying iron protein in the bloodstream) requires an enzyme called ferrochelatase. Ferrochelatase acts like a crane that moves iron and drops it into the center of the heme protein. The crane operator is none other than copper! Without bioavailable copper to serve as that crane operator, we produce kryptopyrroles and defective heme, which causes a reduction in the oxygenation of the blood, and a subsequent loss of both zinc and vitamin B6. Because of how they operate in the body, zinc supplements do not improve these problems, they make them much worse because of their known copper-disrupting properties!

This is why you should not take zinc supplements, including multivitamins (see below) and instead seek to obtain this mineral through your diet.

STOP Taking Molybdenum Supplements

Molybdenum is an essential trace mineral that works in the body to break down proteins and other substances. It is found in a variety of foods, particularly milk, cheese, cereal grains, legumes, kidney beans, nuts, soy products, and dairy, and is primarily stored in the liver. Molybdenum deficiencies are virtually nonexistent, so there is certainly no reason to use molybdenum supplements. Moreover, doing so is detrimental to your health.

Why? Because of what its function is in the body—breaking down proteins. One of which happens to be the vitally important copper-carrying protein I keep calling attention to: ceruloplasmin.

Molybdenum is also a known copper chelator that can create copper deficiency, a scientific fact that was established decades ago. (Phillipo et al, 1987; Bremner et al, 1987; Hurley and Doane, 1989; Moeini et al.1997.) Where this is particularly significant is with ruminant animals, such as cows, sheep, and goats. There are times of the year when the molybdenum and sulfur content of the grass these animals eat is greater, leading to a deficiency of copper that these animals depend upon to make their metabolism work. Studies prove that this occurs because of the higher molybdenum content in the grass, depriving the ruminants from obtaining enough copper. (Gooneratne et al, 1989-Dec, "Review of Copper deficiency and Metabolism of Ruminants." *Canadian Jrl of Animal Science* 69(4): 820-845.)

Excessive levels of molybdenum in humans, which is what you get if you are taking molybdenum supplements, creates this same effect of copper deficiency. In addition, as this copper deficiency occurs, excess molybdenum triggers the formation of a class of toxic compounds called thiomolybdates. Among other health problems, thiomolybdate toxicity in the body, when it reaches a certain level, can cause cancer. Most oncologists are convinced that unbound copper outside of ceruloplasmin is one of the causes of cancer. *They don't understand that they should be asking how and why did the copper get released from ceruloplasmin? Why is copper not enabling the activation of oxygen in the mitochondria? Instead, what they seek to do is eliminate copper, when, instead, arresting the buildup of thiomolybdates is what they should be more focused upon.*

The research clearly shows, "The only way to stop thiomolybdate toxicity through CuMoS4 [copper thiomolybdate] complex formation is to provide a more available form of copper supplement." (https://actavetscand.biomedcentral.com/articles/10.1186/1751-0147-44-S1-P81.) That can't happen if you are taking molybdenum supplements, which are typically found in drugstore and most other multivitamins.

What people don't realize is there are agents in our diet that are causing copper to be released from ceruloplasmin. Then, because of the presence of molybdenum, copper is being gobbled up and excreted. It is not being retained. Ceruloplasmin that is fully loaded with copper, called *holo-ceruloplasmin*, has a lifespan of 144 hours (*six days*). Ceruloplasmin that doesn't have copper, called *apo-ceruloplasmin*, only has a life span of *six hours* Ceruloplasmin is one of the biggest proteins in the body. It contains 1,066 amino acids and six to eight copper atoms, and this protein takes a lot of energy for the body to produce it. If the body has to make it every six hours, as opposed to every six days, you can understand how molybdenum and everything else that cause copper deficiencies create a significant energy loss in the body.

STOP Taking Multivitamins, Multiminerals, and Prenatal Vitamin Products

Despite their popularity, multivitamins, multimineral products, and prenatal vitamin combination supplements, are not designed to optimize bioavailable copper. There are a number of reasons why this is so, none of which you will ever learn from supplement manufacturers and physicians who recommend multivitamin supplements.

The first reason has to do with the fact that all such products are produced from a chemical mixture, or slurry, of ingredients, one of which is iron. Even supplements that claim to be iron-free on the label typically are made from mixtures containing iron. Extra iron consumption, outside of what is found naturally in an Ancestral diet, at any level, is not advisable.

Secondly, these products typically contain vitamin D3, molybdenum, synthetic vitamin C, citrate, and citric *acid*. I've already explained the health risks of vitamin D3 and molybdenum, and will explain why you should never use synthetic ascorbic acid (that is labeled "vitamin C"), as well as any nutrient in citrate form or products containing citric acid, in the next STOP below.

Thirdly, multivitamins and multivitamin products typically contain twice as much calcium as they do magnesium, and up to 15 times as much zinc as they do copper. The dangers of both of these ratios were explained earlier in this chapter.

Fourthly, the B vitamins these products contain are not only synthetic, they are produced as byproducts from the petroleum industry. The very best way to obtain B vitamins is from bee pollen and eating vitamin B-rich foods, such as those recommended in the Ancestral Diet (see Chapter 12).

Finally, and most importantly, the nutrients found in synthetic multivitamin/multimineral products do not work in the same way, or as effectively, in our bodies as do nutrients in food-based formulations. The reason why is very simple. There is a world of difference between a synthetic swill of nutrients produced in a test tube and nutrients that come from organically raised and properly prepared food. Food with soil-derived nutrients, unlike their synthetic analogues, come to us by way of the actions of microbes in the soil that interact with them so that plants, animals, and humans can properly absorb and use them. Synthetic "test tube" nutrients don't have the same energy, frequency, or biology as food-based nutrients. Chemically, they may be similar, but only nutrients that come from the properly mineralized soil that enter our food are truly catalyzing and able to be used inside our bodies, cells and mitochondria the way MTHR Nature intended.

STOP Using Synthetic Forms Of Ascorbic Acid, Citrate, And Citric Acid

Ascorbic acid (apo-vitamin C) is perhaps the most widely known and widely recommended nutrient in the world. As a result, in its most widely used forms (synthetic ascorbic acid and sodium and calcium ascorbate), it is also one of the main culprits in the epidemic of chronic fatigue and disease facing our nation.

I know that may seem heretical, and I'm not asking you to take my word for it.

Instead, please take the words of Carl G. Holmberg and C. B. Laurell, who introduced the scientific community to ceruloplasmin in 1948, eleven years after Albert Szent-Gyorgyi won the Nobel Prize in Physiology or Medicine, in part for being the first person to isolate ascorbic acid and discovering the components and reactions of the citric acid cycle. In their published paper (Isolation of the Copper Containing Protein and a Description of some of its Properties. *Acta Chem Scand.* 2; 1948:550-56), Holmberg and Laurell reported that ascorbic acid is one of the elements capable of breaking down ceruloplasmin, thereby causing it to lose its characteristic blue color and its critical oxidase enzyme functions. Since then, dozens of published studies have repeatedly shown the negative effects of synthetic ascorbic acid on both ceruloplasmin and the enzymatic functions of bioavailable copper.

As an example, consider this 1983 study that appeared in the *American Journal of Clinical Nutrition*, which investigated the effects ascorbic acid had on the copper and ceruloplasmin status of young men. In the study, test subjects consumed 1,500 mg of ascorbic acid each day for a total of 64 days (500 mg with each meal). Blood samples from each of the young men were obtained before the start of the study (day zero), and again on days 28, 52, and 64, and again 20 days after ascorbic acid consumption was discontinued. In their published study, the researchers wrote, *"Serum ceruloplasmin activity was significantly reduced (p less than 0.01) at every data point throughout the ascorbic acid supplementation period. A similar but nonsignificant trend was observed for serum copper. Furthermore, there was a significant increase (p less than 0.01) in serum copper concentration 20 days after the supplementation period. This study confirms that a high ascorbic acid intake is antagonistic to [bioavailable]copper status of men as has been demonstrated in laboratory animals."* (Finley EB, Cerklewski FL. Influence of Ascorbic Acid on Copper Status in Young Adult Men. *Am J Clin Nutr.* Apr 1983;37(4):553-56.)

The bottom line is that all synthetic forms of ascorbic acid act as toxic substances in the human body, and this fact has been known for over 70 years. For at least two generations, coming up on three, we've been propagandized to use synthetic vitamin C supplements while unknowingly destroying our bodies' supply of ceruloplasmin and thus bioavailable copper.

To better understand the significant differences between ascorbic acid and ascorbate compared to real, food-based vitamin C, consider a car. Real vitamin C as it occurs in nature (food-based) is like a complete car that has an engine, a steering wheel, four wheels, and a shell. And in that whole food vitamin C-complex, the "engine" is an enzyme called tyrosinase, which is one of the most important copper-based enzymes in our body. It has two copper atoms inside it, protects us from ultraviolet radiation and is what enables the production of melanin, which is a very important factor for not just our hair color, eye color, and skin color, but is also for energy production.

Compared to the real vitamin C-complex, ascorbic acid and ascorbate are simply the shell of the car, without the engine, nor any other moving parts. We want a car that is complete and dynamic, not a shell of a car that is incapable of moving. The same thing is true in terms of what our bodies want and need—real, fully complexed vitamin C, not the far inferior synthetic form that lacks the key copper atoms that Mother Nature intended us to have access to.

I will discuss the benefits of real vitamin C and the additional reasons why you should stop using ascorbic acid and ascorbate in more detail in Chapter 10. For now, I simply want to add one more reason why you should avoid using synthetic ascorbic acid: Nearly all of it is manufactured from genetically modified corn, and most of it comes from China, which is infamous for its low production standards in the manufacture of nutritional and herbal supplements.

As for why you should avoid both citrate and citric acid, the reason for doing so was discovered by researchers Earl Frieden and Shigemasa Osaki of Florida State University, whose investigations dating back to the mid-1960s clearly demonstrated that citrate suppresses and acts as a natural killer of ceruloplasmin. (Osaki S, McDermott JA, and Frieden E. Citric Acid As The Principle Serum Inhibitor of Ceruloplasmin. *J Biol Chem*. Feb 1964; 239:364-6.)

In order to fully eliminate your intake of synthetic vitamin C, citrate, and citric acid, avoid packaged foods because all three ingredients are commonly found in them. Also, get into the habit of reading food labels, and avoid citrate forms of minerals, including magnesium citrate.

STOP Using High Fructose Corn Syrup (HFCS) And Synthetic Sugars

Consuming high fructose corn syrup and synthetic sugars is one of the worst things you can do for your health. Even conventional physicians with little to no training in nutrition understand that and warn their patients about the dangers of these sweet poisons.

What they likely don't understand or are unaware of, however, is that HFCS and synthetic sugar in all forms block the doorways that allow copper into the body. They prevent dietary copper from being absorbed in the gut and block copper from entering into the cells. That's really all you need to know as to why you should absolutely avoid HFCS and synthetic sugars. However, you must also be on your guard, because, while HFCS isn't used as much as it once was, synthetic sugars still remain quite common as unhealthy additives in many packaged foods and drinks. Ideally, you should avoid these products altogether.

STOP Using Industrialized Omega-6 Oils (e.g. Soybean Oil, Canola Oil, Etc.)

In recent years, an increasing number of scientists and physicians have finally caught up with the fact that industrialized omega-6 oils, such as soybean, canola, safflower, and corn oils, cause rampant inflammation in the body. Yet, the use of such oils still remains widespread, including as additives in many packaged foods, as well as in most commercial breads, mayonnaise, and so forth. They are also widely used in restaurants, especially canola oil, which is probably the worst of the lot.

Omega-6 oils are unsaturated oils and, like saturated oils, they contain essential fatty acids (EFAs). The difference between what makes a fat saturated rather than unsaturated comes down to carbon and hydrogen atoms. All fatty acids are composed of chains of carbon atoms. Each of these carbon atoms can hold up to two hydrogen atoms. Fatty acids in which two hydrogen atoms are attached to each carbon atom make up saturated fats.

Carbon atom chains in fatty acids that are missing one or more hydrogen atoms are found in the unsaturated fats in omega-6 oils, also known as polyunsaturated oils. Fatty acids missing more than two hydrogen atoms in its carbon chain are polyunsaturated, and the more hydrogen atoms missing from its carbon chain, the more polyunsaturated the fatty acid is said to be. This is what makes omega-6 more volatile than saturated oils. *They are much more reactive.* When you start adding iron filings to wheat flour, and you move away from butter and move to corn oil, you've just created a reactive engine. You've got iron reacting with omega-6 oils and stealing hydrogen ions that cause a chain reaction of lipid peroxidation (rusting). That's what initiates oxidative stress. Iron accelerates the mechanism of lipid peroxidation, which is why these oils are so dangerous. And yet they continue to be called "heart healthy." Some within the medical community are starting to recognize the fallacy of that, but it's taken them 70 years to do so.

The other thing that most doctors fail to understand is the effect omega-6 oils have on prostaglandins. Prostaglandins are a group of lipids (fats) found in nearly all human tissues. They are highly reactive, and omega-6 oils can significantly increase this reactivity. As this occurs, the body's healing processes is diminished, inflammation and pain can occur, and overall health is negatively impacted.

What is especially important to understand is that the conversion of arachidonic acid to prostaglandins (PGE2 and PGF2a) is accelerated by the state of copper deficiency (Lampi KJ et al, 1988). Furthermore, the enzyme, cyclooxygenase 2, that triggers this arachidonic acid to prostaglandin reaction, is ramped up in states of copper deficiency (Schuschke DA et al, 2009). And finally, when copper becomes unbound from ceruloplasmin, it, too, is reactive and causes an increase in prostaglandins (PGE2 and PGF2a) (Maddox et al., 1993).

The way to stop these problems is to limit our omega-6 oil intake and to follow the Root Cause Protocol so that we have more bioavailable copper at our disposal.

STOP Using Fluoride (Toothpaste, Tap Water, Etc.)

Fluoride, technically fluorine, is the most reactive element on the planet. Oxygen is the second most reactive element. Adding fluoride to our nation's municipal drinking water was a terrible mistake for many reasons, most especially because combining the two most reactive substances on Earth—fluoride with the oxygen in water—is a perfect recipe for creating oxidative stress. That is reason enough for avoiding drinking tap water and, if possible, showering and bathing in it, since fluoride and other toxic chemicals commonly found in tap water can be absorbed through the skin.

Fluoride also displaces magnesium. This well-established fact was confirmed in a 1995 paper published in the *Journal of the International Society for Fluoride Research*, which stated, *"The toxic effect of fluoride ion plays a key role in acute Mg [magnesium] deficiency. The amount of F [fluoride] assimilated by living organisms constantly increases, and Mg absorption diminishes as a consequence of progressively advancing industrialization."* (Machoy-Mokrzynska A, 1995-Nov, Fluoride-Magnesium Interaction. *J. Int Soc Fluoride Res*;28(4):175-177.) This is the reason why workers in aluminum plants and munitions factories are tested for fluoride toxicity by measuring the amount of magnesium fluoride (MgF) in their bones. The more fluoride you consume and absorb—whether from tap water, toothpaste, fluoridated mouthwashes; it makes no difference—the more you are displacing magnesium from your cells, tissues, blood, and kidneys, as well as your body's metabolic pathways. (Ibid.)

There is also a known impact that fluoride has upon copper and most notably the key complex in the mitochondria, cytochrome c oxidase. Fluoride has proven in study after study to create oxidative stress and kill the ability of the mitochondria to activate oxygen when it is present (Muijers et al, 1994; Fina et al, 2014).

What is especially important to grasp is that fluoride is not just in our drinking water. It also is in dental treatments, and routinely found in prescription medications. Any medication that has the letter "F" in its name, uses fluoride to activate that medication. A case in point is the antibiotic CIPRO (ciprofloxacin), which has a well-earned reputation for ligament ruptures due to its copper chelating abilities that undermines and weakens the copper-dependent enzyme lysyl oxidase, that is central to knitting collagen with elastin, thereby providing tissue integrity. CIPRO is also legendary for causing loss of magnesium.

STOP Using Colloidal Silver As An Antibiotic/ Antimicrobial

In recent years, colloidal silver has become increasingly popular as a so-called natural alternative to antibiotic/antiviral/antifungal drugs due to the many alternative health practitioners who continue to promote its use. While short-term use may provide some benefit, using colloidal silver on a regular basis is a serious mistake.

To understand why, take a look at the periodic table of elements. There, you will find that silver sits right below copper. One of the properties of that class of elements is that the lower elements can displace, or kick out, the higher elements. That's exactly what silver does with copper. Once copper is displaced from the body, you've lost the ability to activate oxygen, and to also deactivate oxidants.

Unlike copper, silver doesn't have a relationship with oxygen. Does it stop infections? Yes, it does. It has known properties that act as a disinfectant, which is all well and good, but when you use colloidal silver, you've lost the mechanism to control the process of oxidative stress in the body. So, although colloidal silver may solve the short-term problem of the infection, what it also does is create metabolic chaos. It is the colloidal form that is so destructive when it comes to destroying bioavailable copper status. But through a quirk of nature, there is a form, called "nano-silver" that does not have the same copper disrupting properties. As you learn more about how the immune system is a function of the vitality of its mitochondria, the need for this "nano-silver bullet" may subside as you regain your homeostasis with the RCP.

There are much better solutions for protecting yourself against infections, the best of which happens to be following the Root Cause Protocol.

STOP Eating Low-Fat, High-Carbohydrate, Processed, Refined Foods

The reason for this last STOP is obvious once you understand the rationale behind each of the previous eleven STOPS. Simply put, the standard Western diet (SWD) of low-fat, high carbohydrate, processed and refined foods, along with unhealthy beverages, is where all of the above risk factors that destroy health and deplete energy converge. People who follow such a diet (most Americans, unfortunately, including many doctors) are eating far too much sugar and unhealthy carbohydrates, and far too many bad sources of oils and fatty acids, and they are not supplying themselves with minerals at the rate and ratios that our bodies need them. As a result, levels of systemic and ongoing oxidative stress within the American populace are through the roof.

America's poor eating habit is one of the primary reasons why the vast majority of people in the United States are chronically fatigued and why we lead the world in the incidences of obesity, diabetes, cancer, heart disease, arthritis, Alzheimer's and dementia, and so many other chronic, serious, degenerative diseases. As Ben Edwards, MD wisely points out, prior to World War II, the United States was number one in terms of its health status in the world. Today, 75 years later, we have one of the lowest health statuses on the planet, and the primary thing that has changed during that time is our diet. He's absolutely right.

Fortunately, you needn't be part of this wholly unhealthy trend. Your dietary habits are something you have complete control over. And once you adopt what I call the Ancestral Diet, which I explain in detail in Chapter 12, you will be well on your way to making the Root Cause Protocol part of your daily life, resulting in improved health and far more energy.

As I wrote as the end of Chapter 6, putting each of the above STOPS into action can go a long way towards making you healthier. To obtain the full range of benefits the Root Cause Protocol provides, however, there are a number of additional steps, which I've termed the RCP **STARTS**, which we also need to adopt. How to do so and in which order is laid out for us in the next chapter.

CHAPTER

8

The STARTS–Putting the Root Cause Protocol Into Practice

"It does not matter how slowly you go as long as you do not stop."

-- Confucius

Once more, allow me to summarize the three key reasons that serve as the underlying rationale for, and foundation of, the Root Cause Protocol. The priority of the RCP is to optimize energy production via magnesium and bioavailable copper:

Bioavailable copper activates oxygen into energy and converts toxic ferrous iron (Fe ++) into the protein-bound ferric iron (Fe +++).

Without enough bioavailable copper, oxygen combines with unbound toxic ferrous iron and they run around the body like a four-year-old with a hammer, causing oxidative stress and systemic inflammation ("rust"), the root cause of fatigue and virtually all health challenges.

Therefore, the priority focus of The Root Cause Protocol is to increase bioavailable copper, which will optimize energy production and minimize oxidative stress and therefore, minimize the magnesium burn rate (MBR). This can be achieved by implementing each of the STOPS and STARTS of the Root Cause Protocol.

This chapter will teach us how to most effectively achieve these ends.

Remember, as soon as the body's tissues cannot produce optimal levels of ATP, the oxygen that is supposed to get activated to make ATP gets diverted and becomes oxidants, aka reactive oxygen species (ROS). As this metabolic conflict builds, the intensity of symptoms builds in equal measure.

Guidelines For Beginning The STARTS

There are three phases to the RCP STARTS, and each element of each phase is listed and explained below. You will also find a complete time table and "roadmap" you can follow as you begin to add each of the STARTS to your daily lifestyle. Keep in mind that these are suggested guidelines only. You do not need to follow all of the STARTS in the exact order as they are laid out in this chapter for the Root Cause Protocol to work for you. Again, please know that these STARTS are available on printable document from the dedicated book website: http://cureyourfatiguebook.com/resources

Many people, when they think of the word protocol, might envision something akin to an airplane pilot going through a pre-flight checklist with exact steps and exact sequences. The Root Cause Protocol is intended to be different from that. *The RCP is about pursuing the right direction, not attaining perfection.* (Please read that again and let it sink in.)

You do NOT have to do every START in the exact right order and dose to begin repairing cellular and mitochondrial dysfunction.

In fact, just quitting the STOPS discussed in Chapter 7 alone will have notable positive impact on your health.

The RCP is a process, not a rigid cookie cutter recipe. Moreover, it is set up so that you can experiment with it and determine for yourself how best to implement it according to your personal experience and evaluation of the health-related improvements you notice as you adopt the RCP. Don't worry about "getting it perfect," just continue moving forward. Begin by stopping today all of the 12 STOPS in Chapter 7. Then slowly begin implementing each of the STARTS, step by step, phase by phase.

One of the most commonly asked questions from people new to the Root Cause Protocol is *"When should I move from the first phase to each of the other two phases?"* The truthful answer is that "it depends." Specifically, it depends upon how well and quickly your body reacts, and then adjusts, to each of the nutrients you will be adding to your daily diet as you progress through the RCP. The "course record" is a woman who implemented all of the STARTS of all three of the phases within a few weeks and experienced dramatic positive changes in her health after only 60 days. On the other hand, there are others who have taken 18 months or longer to adopt all of the STARTS because their bodies needed that much time to detoxify and acclimate to the positive biochemical transformations the RCP triggers. Your mileage will vary. Listen to your body. If you would like personalized help, please consider working with an RCP Consultant who can help you. (See the Resources section for more information.)

Another common question is, *"How long do I need to follow these steps?"* The answer is, ideally, for the rest of your long and healthy life. The Root Cause Protocol is not a diet or other temporary "health fix". It is a *lifestyle program*, one that is designed to always provide you with the important minerals and other nutrients that your body will always need, especially in the face of continued stress. To that end, the STARTS are designed to be followed indefinitely, continually providing you with the key nutrients missing today in the standard Western, highly processed diet, which is laden with so many unhealthy, refined and processed foods, unhealthy fats, and excessive iron fortification. Each of the RCP's phases are additive, meaning that when you begin Phase 2, you should still continue following Phase 1, and continue following Phases 1 and 2 when you begin Phase 3.

Ultimately, The Root Cause Protocol is about education and empowerment. I developed it and wrote this book out of my desire to help us all understand the root cause of our fatigue, which is the triggering event for other health challenges we may presently have. As we implement each of the STARTS in each of the Phases, we will be taking greater and greater control of our health.

The STARTS Of Phase 1: Foundations

There are five STARTS within Phase 1 of the Root Cause Protocol. Again, these STARTS are available on printable document from the dedicated book website: https://cureyourfatiguebook.com/resources The STARTS are as follows:

1) START Taking Trace Mineral Drops

There are two classes of minerals: Macrominerals, and micro, or trace, minerals. In order to function properly, our body needs a daily supply of macrominerals at a dose of at least 100 milligrams (mg) (much higher than that in some cases, such as magnesium).

Trace minerals, which include copper and iodine, are so named because they are needed in amounts of only a few milligrams or micrograms (mcg) per day. Even so, trace minerals are crucial for many functions in the body, including serving as the building blocks for hundreds of enzymes, facilitating numerous biochemical reactions, supporting normal growth and development, maintaining brain health and neurological function, acting as antioxidants, maintaining healthy blood, and playing essential roles in the production and functioning of various hormones.

Like macrominerals, trace minerals are inorganic, meaning they cannot be produced or synthesized by your body. Adding trace minerals to drinking water that you consume each day is the easiest way to ensure that you obtain all of the trace minerals you need. Simply add half a teaspoon of liquid trace minerals to one gallon of water and sip throughout the day. In addition, be sure to use this mineralized water in any recipes that call for water.

Trace mineral drops can be purchased at most health food stores and are also available online. You will find a listing of products and manufacturers of the brands I recommend at the end of this chapter.

2) START Taking The "Adrenal Cocktail"

In addition to not having enough bioavailable copper and magnesium to power their cellular mitochondria, people who suffer from chronic fatigue typically also suffer from what has been termed "adrenal fatigue." Our adrenal glands, which sit atop of our kidneys, regulate production of some 50 hormones, especially cortisol production, as well as the production of another key hormone called aldosterone. Cortisol is focused on protecting potassium status, and aldosterone protects sodium status.

Nutritional deficiencies and the types of chronic stress that we learned about in Chapter 7 can significantly impair adrenal function over time, causing excessive, pro-inflammatory cortisol levels, and a depletion of aldosterone, which, in turn, can deplete potassium levels. The result is persistent fatigue and feelings of "hitting the wall" energetically, and sometimes accompanying anxiety, depression, and other negative emotions. Adrenal fatigue can also lead to poor sleep, making recovery from fatigue even more difficult.

There are a number of do-it-yourself adrenal cocktail recipes. In general, any Adrenal Cocktail recipe should deliver approximately

375 mg of potassium, 460 mg of sodium (salt) in order to support aldosterone production, and 60 mg of whole food vitamin C. The original base recipe is as follows:

4 ounces of organic orange juice. Fresh squeezed is key, and please be sure to avoid commercial orange juice products with added calcium. The vitamin C-complex in orange juice helps to ensure that the minerals noted below get to the liver to then nourish the adrenals.

1/4 tsp of Cream of Tartar (potassium bitartrate). This is an excellent source of potassium. As an alternative, you can use potassium bicarbonate or potassium chloride.

1/4 tsp of fresh ground Redmond's Real Salt or sea salt. This is an excellent source of sodium, plus 90+ other trace minerals.

(Please know that the original source of this recipe was Susan Blackard, NP, ND, PhD, at the Rejuvenation Health Center in Springfield, MO. The following alternatives have been compiled by UBER MAG-pie and RCP enthusiast, Valerie Engh.)

Alternative #1: Replace Cream of Tartar and orange juice with organic coconut water and whole food vitamin C-complex.

8 oz. / 1 cup / 250 mL of coconut water. Be sure to use enough coconut water to ensure you receive 375 mg of potassium.

1/4 tsp of fresh ground Redmond's Real Salt or sea salt.

60 mg of whole food vitamin C-complex.

Alternative #2: Use pure, filtered water and, instead of Cream of Tartar, orange juice, or organic coconut water, use:

1/4 tsp potassium bicarbonate powder. (Prescribed for Life brand is recommended and, again, you want to ensure you receive 375mg of potassium.)

1/4 tsp of fresh ground Redmond's Real Salt or sea salt.

60 mg of whole food vitamin C-complex.

4 oz. of purified water

Alternative #3: Use Cream of Tartar, but use water instead of orange juice or coconut water.

3/4 tsp Cream of Tartar.

1/4 tsp of fresh ground Redmond's Real Salt or sea salt.

60 mg of whole food vitamin C-complex.

4 oz. of purified water.

Substitutions: You may substitute whole food vitamin C-complex for half a freshly squeezed lime or lemon. And you may substitute potassium bicarbonate for potassium gluconate or potassium chloride. Please adjust quantity to ensure you are getting 375mg of potassium.

Instead of using these above DIY recipes, you can also use any of the pre-mixed Adrenal Cocktail products listed below.

Dose: 1 - 2 times per day, best taken at mid-morning and mid-afternoon, as it's better to take the Adrenal Cocktail away from food. Most people start with once per day, and eventually work up to twice per day after several weeks or months, depending on how their body responds. That said, there are some folks who find that they need a third Adrenal Cocktail, often taken just before bed. Again, this in not necessarily a recommendation, but merely sharing the "*in vivo*" experiences of RCP users in the field.

3) START Taking Whole Food Vitamin C-Complex

As Chapter 7 explained, all synthetic versions of ascorbic acid and ascorbate are NOT to be used in the Root Cause Protocol. Whole food, or real, vitamin C-complex, however, is another essential part of the RCP. In addition to the whole food vitamin C-complex you will obtain from the Adrenal Cocktail, I recommend taking 400 mg - 800 mg per day of whole food vitamin C-complex as a supplement. Most people start with 400 mg per day, and eventually work up to 800 mg per day after several weeks or months. Start with the lower level and then work up to the higher level, depending on how your body responds.

4) START Taking Magnesium

"Without enough magnesium, cells simply don't work." This quote by Lawrence M. Resnick, MD, former Professor of Medicine at Weill Cornell Medical School, sums up all you need to know to understand why it is so important that you daily obtain all the magnesium your body needs. If you suffer from fatigue, you can be sure you also suffer from magnesium deficiency, as was discussed in Chapter 3. Let's take a deeper dive so you can more fully appreciate this most essential mineral.

For the past four decades, an average of 2,000 scientific studies per year about the health benefits of magnesium have been published in medical journals around the globe. Sadly, however, for the most part, these studies continue to go unnoticed by the medical community.

This mighty mineral, primarily acting within our cells, is responsible for the proper functioning of approximately 80 percent of the body's metabolic processes. It aids these functions by activating thousands of metabolic pathways in the body, including those responsible for protein, carbohydrate, and fat metabolism. Magnesium also plays a vital role in energy metabolism because it is essential for key steps of anaerobic glycolysis and the Krebs cycle, as well as the stabilization of adenosine triphosphate (Mg-ATP), the cells' main source of energy generation. Magnesium is essential for the production and storage of energy inside each of our 100 trillion cells. That's a lot of ATP, and that's a lot of magnesium, too. An interesting way of understanding the significance of this activity is that we generate our body weight in Mg-ATP each and every day.

Magnesium is also the essential nutrient for muscles, playing a vital role in their proper functioning and, most importantly, their relaxation, so they can be ready for the next contraction. Without magnesium, our muscles simply could not operate the way nature intended.

Magnesium is an absolute for vital, proper heart function. It plays a recognized role in protecting against heart disease, including heart attacks, stroke, and hypertension (high blood pressure), which is clearly documented in hundreds of research studies. This fact seems to be completely unknown to cardiologists, much to the detriment of their patients, and helps to explain why heart disease remains so prevalent in our society—the number one cause of death worldwide, as well as in America for the past 90 years. A comprehensive meta-analysis, published in 2012, brought this point home. The analysis examined previous studies involving more than 241,000 participants and found a "statistically significant inverse association between magnesium intake and risk of stroke." In other words, the less magnesium in your body, the greater your risk for stroke. (Larsson S, et al, 2012, Dietary Magnesium intake and risk of stroke: a meta-analysis of prospective studies. *Am J Clin Nutr*; 95(2): 269-270.)

Additional research has also shown that patients with low magnesium levels have a higher risk of dying of heart disease compared to patients with higher magnesium levels. Research shows that it acts as a natural calcium channel blocker, but without any of the health risks posed by calcium channel blocker drugs (Rosanoff A, Seelig MS, 2004-Oct, Comparison of mechanism and functional effects of Magnesium and statin pharmaceuticals. *J Am Coll Nutr*;23(5):501S-505S. PMID: 15466951), and also helps to prevent the formation of dangerous blood clots (Sheu JR, Hsiao G, et al, 2003-May, Antithrombotic effects of Magnesium sulfate in in vivo experiments. *Int J Hematol*;77(4):414-9. PMID: 12774935). Adequate levels of magnesium also help to regulate blood pressure levels and prevent high blood pressure (Guerrero-Romero F, Rodríguez-Morán M, 2009-Apr, Oral Magnesium supplementation with MgCl significantly reduces blood pressure in diabetic hypertensive adults with hypomagnesaemia. *J Hum Hypertens*;23(4):245-51. Epub 2008 Nov 20. PMID: 19020533), and protects against spasms in the arteries. And, of course, its role in Mg-ATP production is also essential for protecting the heart, since heart muscle cells contain very high concentrations of mitochondria that depend on ATP to do their job. Case in point, it takes one billion Mg-ATP to perform ONE heart beat.

Note: As important as magnesium is for optimal heart function, we must not forget the observations and pioneering research of Jerome L. Sullivan, MD, PhD who introduced the concept of the "Iron-Heart Hypothesis" that we discussed in Chapter 3. Every aspect of magnesium loss noted above is caused by copper-iron dysregulation in the endothelial layer of cells or cardiomyocytes (heart muscle cells). It is this dysregulation that causes increased oxidative stress that then causes magnesium loss in the cells of those tissues. *Heart symptoms are NOT caused by magnesium deficiency, but by a copper deficiency causing iron overload in the tissues of the heart and blood vessels that THEN causes a loss of magnesium. This loss of magnesium is critical, but is a downstream mineral/metabolic event.*

Also important, however, is the magnesium burn rate (MBR) in relation to heart and overall health. The more that stressors impact our lives, the more our body stores of magnesium get depleted (burned up), resulting in a greater degree of oxidative stress that builds up inside our cells. *Again, oxidative stress eats magnesium for lunch!*

Given these and the numerous other benefits magnesium provides, we can see why our need to ensure we are obtaining enough magnesium daily so that our body has an optimal supply to maintain our health and energy in our increasingly stressful and toxic world. The first step to this end, is to regularly consume magnesium-rich foods, but unfortunately that is not enough, in my opinion. Taking daily magnesium supplements are also vitally important.

Magnesium-Rich Foods: Try to eat as many of these magnesium-rich foods (choose organic whenever possible) as you can each day. Please note, though, that it's basically impossible to reach an optimal daily dose of magnesium with food alone. Also, nearly all of these foods also contain calcium. So you cannot rely on food to repair a calcium-magnesium imbalance.

Nuts (Cashews, Brazil, Almonds) [**NOTE:** Almonds and cashews have the same amount of mg/serving, but almonds have six times more calcium per unit of intake.]

Seeds (Sunflower, Pumpkin, Chia, Flax, Hemp)

Dark Leafy Greens (Mustard, Collard, Beet, Chard)

Legumes (Black Beans, Lentils, Chickpeas)

Whole Grains (Oats, Barley, Buckwheat, Quinoa)

Fish (Halibut, Salmon, Mackerel)

Dark chocolate, unsweetened cocoa/cacao

Magnesium Supplements: The optimal dose of "elemental" magnesium is 5 mg per pound of body weight, per day (or 10 mg of magnesium per kilogram of body weight, per day). So, if you weigh 200 lbs (90 kg), your eventual goal is 1,000 mg per day using magnesium-rich foods and oral magnesium supplements and/or topical magnesium. This dosing formula was originally created by Mildred S. Seelig, MD, MPH, who is considered by many to have been the foremost authority on magnesium. You will most likely need to build up to this dose over several months, based upon bowel tolerance. Choose A) a form of magnesium malate, B) a form of magnesium glycinate, and C) a form of topical magnesium lotion or oil from the recommended products listed at the end of this chapter.

Dosing and Timing: We recommend that magnesium supplementation be at 5 mgs/pound or 10 mgs/kilogram body weight. That is based on steady state levels of stress. Should the level of stress increase significantly, please add more to the mix. Please take in divided doses throughout the day. Some forms are more energizing (malate) and others are more relaxing (glycinate), so choose the form that works best for you.

Magnesium lotion or oil, one application in the evening. (**Note:** Magnesium lotion is generally better tolerated on the skin than magnesium oil, but oil can be mixed into water for a good foot or bath soak, so it's difficult to recommend one over the other. Choose the one that best suits you. As an alternative to using magnesium lotion or oil, you can also use Epsom salt to make a magnesium-rich foot or bath soak.)

5) START Eating grass-fed organic beef liver

It's hard to emphasize the importance of this one source of food that is overflowing with life-enhancing nutrients that our Ancestors took for granted. It is among the richest sources of bioavailable copper (a healthy liver has twice as much copper as iron, contrary to your beliefs), choline, retinol, hyaluronic acid, to name but a few. And as we'll see in the next Phase, we'll be revisiting this food for its legendary sources of real B vitamins. The key to this food, however, is eating it from cows allowed to eat their natural diet of grass.

What may come as a surprise is to learn that grass has vastly more beta-carotene (precursor to retinol) than carrots and in similar fashion, vastly more real vitamin C than oranges! And while you may find the taste offensive, I'm confident that this is the result of eating grain-fed and not grass-fed beef liver. It is a blockbuster component of the RCP and I encourage you to give it a fair trial. As we'll see, there is also an option of ingesting desiccated beef liver for those that can't find the real deal or can't bring themselves to actually eat it. Also, we'll revisit this key food as an important source of real B vitamins.

The STARTS Of Phase 2: Supporting Nutrients

How long you remain only on Phase 1 of the RCP depends on you. So long as you continue to gain benefit from it, stay on it. Once you feel that your gains have plateaued, you will be ready to move into Phase 2, which consists of five additional STARTS that you will add to the five STARTS of Phase 1. These additional STARTS are easy to do and simply involves adding what we call MTHR Nature sources of foods that are rich in B vitamins, wholefood vitamin E, Boron and everyone's favorite, Cod Liver Oil (CLO).

6) START Eating Organic Whole Foods

The goal of this START step is for you to start being more aware of what you eat. Instead of processed and packaged foods, and the other foods and beverages included in the STOPS chapter, aim for fresh, locally-grown, organic, seasonal foods, including grass-fed meats, pasture-raised poultry, coldwater, wild-caught seafood, and a plentiful supply of organic (if possible) fresh fruits and vegetables, while limiting or completely eliminating your intake of grains and other high-carbohydrate foods.

In general, you will be following what I call an Ancestral Diet, with a mix of high fat, moderate protein, and low carbohydrates. But do not think about this as a "diet," per se, and don't get hung up on trying to eat perfectly. Remember, the RCP is about direction, not perfection. (You will find more guidelines for incorporating the Ancestral Diet into your lifestyle in Chapter 12.)

7) START Taking MTHR Nature's Sources for B Vitamins

B vitamins (collectively known as the B-complex) play many important roles in your body, including supporting the health of your brain, eyes, intestines, liver, muscle, and skin. Additionally, B vitamins are essential for proper energy production and metabolism, and play an essential role in sleep because of the sedative effect they have on the nerves and their ability to help the human body cope with stress. Being water-soluble, they cannot be stored by our body, and can quickly be depleted, especially during times of stress. There are many B vitamins, eight of which have been designated as important for your health: B1, B2, B3, B5, B6, B7, B9, and B12.

Note: When supplementing with vitamin B products, be sure to ONLY USE food-based vitamin B supplements. This is vitally important, because most vitamin supplements are synthetic and many are made from coal tar derivatives.

The Best MTHR Nature Sources of B Vitamins: Each of the above B vitamins work best in combination with all of the other B vitamins. Taken together, they provide synergistic health benefits that are greater than the benefits they can provide separately on their own. That is why it is best for you to obtain a complete daily supply of B vitamins from natural food sources, NOT synthetic vitamin B formulas, which, again, are made from coal tar derivatives, a fact few people are aware of.

The three best food sources of B vitamins are bee pollen, stabilized rice bran, and grass-fed beef liver. I recommend that you make all three part of your daily RCP routine.

Bee Pollen: If possible, obtain bee pollen from local, organic bee farms in your area. If that is not possible, then choose one of the recommended brands below. Take ½ - 1 teaspoon daily at breakfast. By the way, a bee produces approximately one teaspoon of bee pollen in six weeks. The lifespan of a bee is also six weeks, so let us all "bee" grateful for their work!

Caution: Some people who are allergic to bee stings, are also allergic to honey and bee pollen, which can cause anaphylactic shock for such individuals. Anaphylactic shock, if not treated in time, can be fatal. Do NOT use bee pollen if you are allergic, or suspect you are, to bee stings or bee products.

Stabilized Rice Bran: Stabilized rice bran is derived from under the hull of rice. In its stabilized form, it is one of the most nutritionally rich foods in the world, containing not only B vitamins, but also numerous other vitamins, minerals (including magnesium), amino acids, and essential fatty acids. It is also a good source of both soluble and insoluble fiber. A daily dose is between one and two teaspoons, taken away from food. Ideal times are right before you go to bed at night, or right after you get up in the morning, at least half an hour before breakfast.

Grass-Fed Beef Liver, or Beef Liver Supplements: A key critical fact that underscores the importance of eating beef liver: In 1934, Drs. George H. Whipple, George R. Minot, and William P. Murphy were awarded the Nobel Prize in Physiology or Medicine for their discovery that beef liver could prevent and reverse anemia, as well as pernicious (B12) anemia. Simply put, beef liver is one of the best foods you can eat to boost your energy levels. Not only is it rich in B vitamins, it also provides a healthy dose of real vitamin A. I recommend that you eat four to six ounces of organic, grass-fed beef liver once a week or more, if you can properly source it. If not, please choose one of the recommended brands of Desiccated Beef Liver Supplements listed below and work up to taking 3,000 mg each day, dividing the dose to 1,500 mg taken with breakfast and dinner.

8) START Taking Whole Food Vitamin E-Complex

Whole food vitamin E-complex is another important antioxidant that neutralizes free-radical damage. Vitamin E has a recognized and unique ability to stop lipid peroxidation, the originating source of oxidation in most tissues. It is also a powerful immune-enhancing nutrient, primarily because of its ability to increase levels of the interferon (IFN-y) and interleukin (IL's), two biochemicals that are required by the immune system to prevent and fight off infections. In addition, vitamin E is key for synthesizing CoQ10 (aka, ubiquinone), a key player in energy production in the mitochondria.

Adequate vitamin E levels in the body can help protect against a variety of other conditions, as well, including certain types of cancer, respiratory conditions, various eye problems (including macular degeneration and vision issues related to diabetes), prostate enlargement, osteoarthritis, and sunburn. It has also shown promise for preventing Alzheimer's disease and dementia. To obtain all of these benefits, it is important that you only use whole food vitamin E-complex, not the synthetic versions that typically only contain alpha-tocopherol.

Dosage: Take one serving daily with lunch. Dosages vary between each recommended product, but a typical suggested dose of whole food vitamin E-complex is 400 IU each day.

(**Caution:** Please be aware that vitamin E, like CLO, has a natural propensity to thin the blood.)

9) START Taking Boron

Boron is a mineral that plays many vitally important roles in the body's metabolic functions. Its two most important roles lie in its ability to bind up oxygen and to help regulate iron. Thus, boron plays a key role in STOPing oxidative stress.

Boron is also essential for the growth and maintenance of bone, preventing arthritis and osteoporosis, and aiding in wound healing. It also helps regulate how the body uses estrogen, testosterone, and vitamin D, and boosts magnesium absorption. In addition, boron protects against oxidative stress in a number of important ways. It reduces levels of inflammatory biomarkers, such as high-sensitivity C-reactive protein (hs-CRP) and tumor necrosis factor α (TNF-α), and raises levels of antioxidant enzymes, such as superoxide dismutase (SOD), catalase, and glutathione peroxidase. Boron has also been shown to help prevent oxidative stress caused by heavy metals and other environmental toxins, including those found in commercial pesticides.

This versatile nutrient also helps improve the brain's electrical activity, cognitive performance, and short-term memory, including among the elderly, and acts as a natural anticancer agent (Pizzorno, L, 2015-Aug, Nothing boring about boron. *Integr Med (Encinitas)*; 14(4): 35–48).

A typical daily dose is between 1,000 to 3,000 mg taken with breakfast.

As another option, you can take a "boron bath" using 20 Mule Team Borax or a similar brand, added to bath water, along with Epsom salt and baking soda.

10) START Taking Cod Liver Oil

Cod liver oil (CLO) is a wonderful source of naturally occurring real vitamin A (as retinol), which is crucial for enabling the synthesis of bioavailable copper, along with the thousands of other metabolic activities that are only enabled by real vitamin A. The omega-3s in CLO are also beneficial, but the naturally occurring vitamin A is what we're really seeking to get.

For adults, start slow and build up to a dose of CLO that delivers 900 mcg /3,000 IU of vitamin A per day. For children, the Recommended Daily Intake (RDI) for vitamin A begins at 400 mcg /1,333 IU and increases to 700 mcg /2,333 IU as they age. Lactating mothers require up to 1,300 mcg /4,333IU, as lactation drains the mother's retinol reserves during the course of breast feeding. It is recommended that you take all of your cod liver oil each day with breakfast.

(**Caution:** Like other oils that contain omega-3 essential fatty acids, CLO has a natural propensity to thin the blood, and its use should be monitored if you are currently taking blood thinner medications.)

The STARTs of Phase 3

In Phase 3 of the RCP, you will be adding three other elements to the STARTS of Phases 1 and 2: taurine, silica/diatomaceous earth, and food sources of iodine.

11) START Taking Taurine

Taurine is a sulfur-based amino acid. It is not considered an essential amino acid because the body can manufacture it from methionine.

However, many people lack cysteine oxidase, the enzyme necessary for this conversion, as well as enough vitamin A and vitamin B6, which are also necessary for this process. (Given that most oxidases are copper dependent, might this be why people lack this pivotal enzyme?)

Taurine is essential for the developing brain and overall brain function. In addition, it stabilizes the electrical charge on cells, helps maintain a regular heartbeat, assists in fat absorption, boosts immunity by aiding white blood cell function, and acts as an antioxidant. The best food sources of taurine are sea foods, especially clams, mussels, and scallops.

A good daily dose of supplemental taurine is 500 mg taken with food at dinner time.

12) START Taking Silica/Diatomaceous Earth

Silica is a mineral in the body that is abundant when we are young, but rapidly declines as we age. It is also water-soluble, so it needs to be replaced on a daily basis. It plays many important roles in the body, including maintaining healthy cholesterol and blood pressure levels, improving digestive function, and aiding in the production of energy. In addition, silica helps to prevent and eliminate intestinal worms and parasites.

Food-grade diatomaceous earth, or DE, is composed of 90 percent silica. DE is formed from the fossilized remains of hard-shelled algae called diatoms. In addition to supplying your body with silica, DE, because of its mildly abrasive properties, has also been shown to aid in the elimination of molds, mucus, fungi, and toxic heavy metals such as mercury from the gastrointestinal tract.

When supplementing with DE, start with ⅛ teaspoon mixed with water, then increase gradually to one teaspoon per day, taken either in the morning or at night, away from both food and other supplements, including rice bran. Also be sure to take it away from any medications your doctor may have prescribed for you. You may find that alternating between DE and stabilized rice bran every other day, usually right before bedtime, works best for you.

13) START Taking Iodine from food sources

Iodine is essential for the proper function of the thyroid gland. In addition, your body's trillions of cells contain and use iodine in order to carry out their many functions. The greatest concentration of iodine in the body is within the endocrine system because iodine is necessary for the production of all of your body's hormones. Within this system, by far the highest concentrations of iodine are found in the thyroid gland. But many other parts of a healthy body also contain large amounts of iodine, including, in women, the mammary glands of the breast. In fact, next to the thyroid gland, breasts serve as one of the female body's primary iodine storage sites. That's because iodine is necessary for proper breast development and function, as well as the maintenance of the breasts' shape and structure.

Iodine deficiency affects nearly all Americans today, due to a variety of factors, such as industrial farming techniques that have depleted croplands of their iodine content, diets lacking in ocean fish or sea vegetables such as kelp, diets that are high in breads and pasta, vegetarian and vegan diets, low-salt diets (salt contains iodine), and the introduction of various chemicals in our food supply and environment, especially halide chemicals such as bromine, a common ingredient used by the baking industry, and fluoride and chloride, both commonly found in our drinking water. Halide chemicals interfere with the body's ability to store and use iodine.

Prerequisite: Before beginning iodine supplements, your RBC magnesium and RBC selenium need to be at optimal levels. (Please refer to Ideal Values for Lab Tests in Chapter 7.) Until then, add iodine-rich foods to your diet, such as kelp and other types of seaweed (all of which also provide selenium), scallops, cod, cranberries, etc.

Once your RBC magnesium and selenium levels are in the ideal values range, you can take one serving of supplemental iodine per day if you choose. Dosages vary between each recommended product listed below, but, similar to whole food vitamin E, the goal is to ensure you are getting some amount of iodine from a whole food source each day. The specific amount is not particularly important.

A Suggested Daily Schedule For All 3 Phases of the Root Cause Protocol

Now that you know and understand each of the STARTS in Phases 1, 2, and 3 of the RCP, let's look at a suggested daily schedule, or timetable, you can use each day to most effectively implement them. The following guidelines provides you with the information you need in order to do so, including each of the supplements you require for each of the phases, as well as the times in which to take them. For those interested in a printable schedule, please go the dedicated book website: **https://cureyourfatiguebook.com/resources**

Throughout the Day

Trace Mineral Drops ~1/2 tsp (mix w/ gallon of water to sip on throughout the day) - Phases 1-3

With Breakfast

Magnesium Malate ~200mg - Phases 1-3

Cod Liver Oil ~900mcg / 3,000 IU - Phases 1-3

Bee Pollen ~½ - 1 tsp - beginning with Phase 2

Beef Liver ~1,500mg - beginning with Phase 1

Boron ~1 - 3mg - Phase 3

Iodine ~ 1 serving - Phase 3

Mid-Morning (away from food)

Adrenal Cocktail 1 serving (mix in OJ or water) - Phases 1-3

Whole Food Vitamin C-complex ~400mg - Phases 1-3

With Lunch

Magnesium Malate ~200mg - Phases 1-3

Whole Food Vitamin E Complex ~ 1 serving - Phases 1-3

Beef Liver ~1,500mg - beginning with Phase 1

Mid-Afternoon (away from food)

Adrenal Cocktail 1 serving (mix in OJ or water) - Phases 1-3

Whole Food Vitamin C-complex ~400mg - Phases 1-3

With Dinner

Taurine ~500mg, - Phase 3

Evening

Magnesium Glycinate ~200mg - Phases 1-3

Topical Magnesium 1 application - Phases 1-3

Right before bed, or first thing in the morning (away from food)

Rice Bran ~1 - 2 tsp - beginning with Phase 2

Diatomaceous Earth ~½ - 1 tsp - Phase 3.

Recommended Handbook

To support this process of adopting these recommended changes, we have developed a user-friendly **RCP Handbook** that is designed to support the adoption of these STOPS & STARTS, as well as provide additional explanation for their importance. This **RCP HANDBOOK** is routinely updated and is available at the RCP website: https://therootcauseprotocol.com/handbook-download/

Recommended Product Brands

I have found the following product brands to be the best sources of the nutritional products you will require for each of the RCP STARTS, based on their high quality and the testing they undergo to ensure their purity. They are available in the US and worldwide, unless noted otherwise.

Please NOTE: for the most complete and accurate listing of recommended products, please direct your attention to https://therootcauseprotocol.com/rcp-product-directory/ We update this listing regularly and strongly recommend drawing from this online directory of products that we endorse.

For those that are interested in the convenience of RCP Product Kits, there are several sets that are available from which to choose on the RCP website product directory.

Trace Minerals

Aussie Trace Minerals (JigsawHealth.com, SeaMineral.com)

Anderson's Sea M.D. Concentrated Mineral Drops (Amazon.com, getsmidge.com.

MineralResourcesInt.com/sea-m-d, RadiantLifeCatalog.com)

Concentrace Trace Mineral Drops (TraceMinerals.com, Amazon. com, iHerb.com, VitaCost.com)

Amena's Daily Boost (Available in Australia at Amenas.com.au)

Ancient Lakes Ionic Magnesium "Bitterns" (AustralianPureMagnesium.com, in Australia at AncientLakes Magnesium.com, in the UK/EU at TreatMeNiceUK.com)

Adrenal Cocktail Mixes

Jigsaw Adrenal Cocktail + Whole Food Vitamin C-complex (Available as a powder in single serving packets or jar; or as capsules; or as a mix it yourself kit at JigsawHealth.com, getsmidge.com, AustralianPureMagnesium.com, Amazon.com; in Australia at NaturallyReplenish.com.au, AncientLakesMagnesium.com; in Australia and Singapore at KimiKimOrganics.com.au; in the UK/EU at DetoxPeople.eu, TreatMeNiceUK.com) Optional: Adrenal Support Ashwaganda (iHerb.com, GaiaHerbs.com)

Whole Food Vitamin C-Complex

Jigsaw Adrenal Cocktail + Whole Food Vitamin C-complex (JigsawHealth.com as a powder in single serving packets or jar; or as capsules. In addition to containing the ingredients for the Adrenal Cocktail, this formula also contains 400 mg of whole food vitamin c-complex as acerola per serving.)

Ama Fruits Acerola Powder (This is included in Corganic's Adrenal Cocktail Kit as getsmidge.com and is sold separately at AmaFruits.com.)

Organic Camu Camu Powder (Amazon.com, iHerb.com, VitaCost.com, NavitasOrganics.com; in Australia and Singapore at KimiKimOrganics.com.au)

Ancient Lakes Pure Kakadu Plum Whole Food Vitamin C (Available as a powder or capsules in the US at AustralianPureMagnesium.com; in Australia at AncientLakesMagnesium.com; in the UK/EU at TreatMeNiceUK.com)

Innate Response Vitamin C-400 (Available as tablets only at InnateResponse.com, iHerb.com, Amazon.com. Ignore the "ascorbic acid" on the label as I've confirmed with the company that this is due to a regulatory issue and this product is indeed from whole foods only.)

Pure Synergy's Pure Radiance C (PureFormulas.com, Amazon. com, iHerb.com, VitaCost.com)

Magnesium Products

Oral Magnesium Malate

Jigsaw MagSRT (B-Free) (time-release tablets; 500 mg of magnesium malate per serving) (JigsawHealth.com; in Canada at Promedics.com; in Australia at NaturallyReplenish.com; in Australia and Singapore at KimiKimOrganics.com; in the UK/EU at DetoxPeople.eu

Jigsaw MagPure Malate (in capsules, providing 100 mg of magnesium malate per serving and available through the same websites as Jigsaw MagSRT above.)

Organic 3, Inc. Wake Up Maggie (200 mg of magnesium as malate, orotate, and taurinate, plus boron, a magnesium co-factor, per scoop of powder) (Organic3.com, getsmidge.com)

Oral Magnesium Glycinate

Jigsaw Mag Now (provides 200 mg of magnesium glycinate plus potassium bicarbonate, a magnesium co-factor, per scoop of powder; available in single serving packets or jars) (JigsawHealth. com, Amazon.com; in Australia at NaturallyReplenish.com; in Australia and Singapore at KimiKimOrganics.com; in the UK/EU at DetoxPeople.eu)

Jigsaw MagPure Glycinate (provides 50 mg of magnesium glycinate per serving capsule) (JigsawHealth.com, Amazon.com; in Australia at NaturallyReplenish.com; in Australia and Singapore at KimiKimOrganics.com; in the UK/EU at DetoxPeople.eu)

Organic 3, Inc. Goodnight Maggie (provides 100 mg of magnesium as bisglycinate chelate and oxide per capsule) (Organic3.com, getsmidge.com)

Doctor's Best Magnesium (Bisglycinate) (DrBVitamins.com. Amazon.com, iHerb.com, VitaCost.com)

Pure Encapsulations Magnesium Glycinate (provides 120 mg magnesium glycinate per capsule a negligible amount of ascorbyl palmitate, a form of synthetic vitamin C) (PureEncapsulations. com, Amazon.com

Topical Magnesium Lotion or Oil

Health and Wisdom (Oil) (Health-and-Wisdom.com, Amazon. com, iHerb.com, VitaCost.com)

Ancient Minerals (Lotion or Oil) (Ancient-Minerals.com, JigsawHealth.com, EnviroMedica.com, Amazon.com)

DermaMag (Oil) (available at DermaMag.com, Amazon.com)

Mo' Maggie (Lotion) (MoNatural.com)

Malle's Magnesium Oil (TheMagnesiumCo.com, getsmidge.com, Amazon.com)

Ancient Lakes Magnesium Oil (AustralianPureMagnesium.com, in Australia at AncientLakesMagnesium.com, in the UK/EU at TreatMeNiceUK.com)

Other Magnesium Alternatives Links

Epsom Salt (for a bath or foot soak) (Available at most local drugstores)

Cod Liver Oil (CLO)

Rosita Real Foods Extra Virgin Cod Liver Oil (Available as liquid and capsules. For liquid, one serving is 3,900 IU. For capsules, take 7 capsules to reach 3,000 IU.) (Available worldwide at RositaRealFoods.com, EVCLO.com; in the US at getsmidge.com, PerfectSupplements.com, RadiantLifeCatalog.com, Amazon.com)

Jigsaw Alaskan Cod Liver Oil (5 soft gels is 975mcg/3,250 IU; 1 soft gel is 195 mcg/650 IU) (JigsawHealth.com, Amazon.com; in Australia at NaturallyReplenish.com; in Australia and Singapore at KimiKimOrganics.com; in the UK/EU at DetoxPeople.eu)

Supplement Facts label. (NordicNaturals.com; iHerb.com. Amazon. com. VitaCost.com; in Australia at NaturallyReplenish.com)

Whole Food Vitamin E-Complex

Life Extension Gamma E Mixed Tocopherols & Tocotrienols (LifeExtension.com, JigsawHealth.com, iHerb.com, Amazon.com, Vitacost.com)

Standard Process Wheat Germ Oil (StandardProcess.com, Amazon.com)

Juka's Organic Red Palm Oil (JukasOrganic.com, getsmidge.com, Amazon.com)

Nutiva Organic Red Palm Oil (Store.Nutiva.com, Amazon.com)

Purely-E (NorthAmericanHerbsAndSpice.com, Amazon.com)

Bee Pollen

(Available in USA; shipping bee pollen internationally has proven to be a problem for some as it may get seized by customs. So again, look for local and organic sources.)

Greenbow Organic Bee Pollen (GreenbowUS.com, JigsawHealth.com, Amazon.com)

Honey Pacifica Bee Pollen (HoneyPacifica.com, getsmidge.com, Amazon.com)

Stakich Bee Pollen (Stakich.com, Amazon.com)

Stabilized Rice Bran

NOW Foods Stabilized Rice Bran (NowFoods.com, JigsawHealth. com, Amazon.com, iHerb.com, VitaCost.com)

Grass-Fed Beef Liver, or Beef Liver Tablets

(For grass-fed beef liver, try to find a local supplier. Beef liver tablets are available in USA; shipping beef liver tablets internationally has proven to be a problem for some as shipments may get seized by customs.)

Perfect Desiccated Liver Capsules (PerfectSupplements.com, JigsawHealth.com; Amazon.com)

Organic 3 Freeze-Dried Beef Liver Capsules (Available worldwide at Organic3.com; in the US at getsmidge.com)

Enviromedica Pasteurized Beef Liver Capsules (US and New Zealand) (Enviromedica.com, Amazon.com)

Ancestral Grass-Fed Beef Liver Capsules (US and New Zealand) (AncestralSupplements.com, Amazon.com)

Pete Evans Grass-Fed Beef Liver Capsules (US and Australia) (Amazon.com, PeteEvans.com, GelatinAustralia.com.au)

Radiant Life Desiccated Liver Capsules (RadiantLifeCatalog.com)

Silica/Diatomaceous Earth

KVL Lab Food-Grade Diatomaceous Earth (available at KVLab. com, JigsawHealth.com) Lumino Food-Grade Diatomaceous Earth (available at LuminoFoodGradeDE.com, getsmidge.com, Amazon.com)

Boron

Trace Minerals Research Ionic Boron (This is a liquid drop formula, and while you do want to limit citric acid intake, the amount used in this formula is miniscule and therefore, negligible.)

(TraceMinerals.com, JigsawHealth.com, VitaCost.com)

Organic 3, Inc. Boron Glycinate (powder) (Organic3.com, getsmidge.com)

Taurine

Douglas Labs Taurine (capsules) (DouglasLabs.com, JigsawHealth. com, Amazon.com

Pure Encapsulations Taurine (capsules) (PureEncapsulations.com, Amazon.com)

NOW Foods Taurine (capsules) (NowFoods.com, iHerb.com, Amazon.com), VitaCost.com)

Iodine

Oregon's Wild Harvest Kelp (capsules) (available at OregonsWildHarvest.com, JigsawHealth.com, Amazon.com, iHerb.com, VitaCost.com)

Seagreen's Iodine+ Organic Dried Seaweed (capsules) (available at SeagreensOnline.com, getsmidge.com. Amazon.com)

RCP PRODUCT KITS

For your convenience, several companies in various regions have created RCP Product Kits.

Jigsaw Health (USA & Worldwide; JigsawHealth.com)

RCP Phase 1 Kit - 2 month supply.

RCP Phase 2 Kit - 2 month supply.

RCP Phase 3 Kit - 2 month supply.

GetSmidge.com (USA & Worldwide; formerly known as getsmidge.com)

RCP Starter Kit (including cod liver oil as softgels) - 1 month supply.

RCP Starter Kit (including cod liver oil as liquid) - 1 month supply.

Naturally Replenish (Australia; NaturallyReplenish.com.au) - All of the RCP products in one kit.

KimiKim Organics (Australia & Singapore; KimiKimOrganics. com.au) RCP Mineral Balance Kit - Most of the RCP products in one kit.

RCP Mineral Balance Medium Kit - Some of the RCP products in one kit.

RCP Mineral Balance Basic Kit - Several of the RCP products in one kit.

Ancient Lakes Magnesium (Australia, EU, USA;)

Sample Packs & Bundles (Australia; AustralianPureMagnesium. com) - Various RCP products.

Sample Packs & Bundles (UK & EU; TreatMeNiceUK.com) - Various RCP products.

Sample Packs & Bundles (USA; AncientLakesMagnesium.com) - Various RCP products.

Detox People (EU; DetoxPeople.eu)

RCP Phase 1 - 2 month supply.

To C and D Or Not To C and D

"A vitamin is a substance that makes you ill if you don't eat it."

– Albert Szent-Gyorgyi, Nobel Laureate (1937)

"You take the healthiest diet in the world, if you gave those people vitamins, they would be twice as healthy. So vitamins are valuable."

– Robert Atkins, MD

I can think of no other nutritional supplements that are more commonly recommended by nutritionally-oriented physicians and other health practitioners than vitamin C and vitamin D. Nor do I know of any other nutrients, except for iron, that can cause such harm as these two nutrients can and do when consumed in their synthetic forms (ascorbic acid/ascorbate and vitamin D3). Going forward, unless specifically noted, when I say "vitamin C," I am specifically referring to REAL vitamin C-complex, and NOT ascorbic acid. When I say "vitamin D," I am referring to the storage form of this hormone, 25(OH)D3, and NOT supplemental-D that comes from a bottle.

I briefly discussed the harm that synthetic C and D can cause and why they should be avoided in Chapter 7. In this chapter, I am going to provide more information that will explain the myths and misconceptions surrounding both of these all-too-popular supplements.

Let me begin with this truth: Try as we might, we humans simply are not capable of improving upon what nature has already provided us with to sustain our health and well-being. That fact alone explains why whole food vitamin C-complex and vitamin D obtained by sunlight and in food are far superior and safer than synthetic vitamin C and D formulations made from test tubes in a lab.

Then let me add this truth: Neither synthetic vitamin C nor synthetic vitamin D will make you sick if you don't consume them. Therefore, according to Szent-Gyorgyi, neither of them can be considered real vitamins (see his opening quote above). Please take a moment and let that observation sink in.

Let's take a deeper dive to look more closely at the myths that keep both synthetic supplements popular among doctors and the public alike.

C-anceling the Ascorbic Acid/Ascorbate Myth

"When you meet with a fact opposed to a prevailing theory, you should adhere to the fact and abandon the theory, even when the latter is supported by great Authority and generally accepted."

– Claude Bernard, MD (1813 – 1878) Founder of
Scientific Method in Medicine

If you only remember one thing from all of the information I am sharing with you in this section, let it be this: Synthetic ascorbic acid/ascorbate is not the same thing as whole food vitamin C-complex, and, unlike whole food vitamin C-complex, which is absolutely essential for good health, synthetic ascorbic acid most definitely is not!

As far as I'm concerned, there is no greater medical or nutritional lie on this planet than that perpetrated on humanity about synthetic vitamin C. This one deception has done more to catabolize (break down) human metabolism than any other dietary recommendation. Proponents of and apologists for this synthetic vitamin may claim that the research into it and whole food vitamin C-complex is "conflicted" and "confusing." That is simply not true. There is no confusion. The natural form of whole food vitamin C-complex found throughout nature has the tyrosinase enzyme at its core. Synthetic vitamin C does not. The tyrosinase enzyme has two copper atoms at its core. This is a scientific fact and not confusing. Lack of the tyrosinase enzyme in our diets has led to a tsunami of oxidative stress that is enabling the "rusting out" of humanity.

Nor is the tyrosinase enzyme all that synthetic vitamin C is lacking. It also lacks the polyphenols rutin and the flavanone glycoside hesperidin (sometimes referred together as "vitamin P"), vitamin K, and factor J (choline), all of which are found in whole food vitamin C-complex, and, along with tyrosinase, are essential co-factor nutrients that work synergistically with ascorbigen, the natural form of L-ascorbic acid that whole food vitamin C-complex also contains. Without these essential co-factors, L-ascorbic cannot be absorbed, which is why 90 percent of synthetic vitamin C supplements are rapidly excreted by the body soon after they are consumed. That should suffice to prove that the human body does not want synthetic vitamin C!

A leading authority on plant stem cell research and embryonic phytochemistry is Dominique Richard. *"Ascorbic acid is not a vitamin,"* he states, *"and I suspect that many other supplements out there, full of synthetic analogues cannot duplicate actual vitamins, since they are severely lacking, as is the case in replacing the [natural] vitamin C-complex with [synthetic] ascorbic acid. Ascorbic acid is also ten times more acidic than the naturally occurring vitamin C-complex."* That fact, alone, should get us to sit up and take notice of the profoundly different chemical properties between these two substances. It is this intensely acidic pH that blocks copper's absorption, alters the structure of ceruloplasmin, and increases the absorption—but NOT mobilization—of iron in the cells and tissues of our body.

He adds that man-made synthetic ascorbic acid analogues lack therapeutic benefits, including against the common cold, because, "they are Fractionated = Synthetic = Crystalline = Unnatural. Natural plant-source vitamins are enzymatically alive. Manmade synthetic vitamins analogues are void of enzymatic activity and work like that of a drug. Most sources equate vitamin C with ascorbic acid, as though they were one within the same thing... Ascorbic acid by itself is a weak antioxidant when not part of the full-spectrum vitamin C-complex composition." (Richard D, 2016-Aug 4, Quantitative Analysis of Vitamin C-Complex Found In Embryonic Plant Extracts.)

As Professor Richard also points out, the body requires whole food vitamin C-complex in order to form collagen in bones, cartilage, and muscle, and to maintain the integrity, strength, and flexibility of blood vessels. It is also of particular importance to the adrenal glands, which Richard says "have an enormous need for vitamin C-complex like no other glands." One of the primary functions of the adrenal glands is to act as our body's "energy reservoir." They play a vital role in supplying us with energy and for helping our body cope with stress. It is estimated that as much as 95 percent of the body's stores for real vitamin C-complex are found in our adrenal glands.

Moreover, according to Professor Richard, "The vitamin C-complex is so much more important than ascorbic acid [for] the armor of the lymphocytes. Lymphocytes without the full spectrum vitamin C-complex will inevitably be impotent, fail to function, and be unable to fight off infectious organisms. The potency of lymphocytes is also linked to copper, the trace mineral found at the core of the tyrosinase enzyme activity. Organic copper, functioning as the tyrosinase enzyme, [is] the most active factor of the vitamin C-complex.

"Scientific research has shown that a relationship exists between ineffective lymphocytes and copper deficiency. These lymphocytes that lack copper, as well as the ability to kill pathogens, may actually be lacking the entire vitamin C-complex, which contains copper. Such ideas are ignored because vitamin C is not detected in lymphocytes. Why isn't vitamin C recognized on the lymphocyte? Well, researchers recognize vitamin C as ascorbic acid, which is shed in the human body and not taken up by the lymphocyte with the rest of the C-complex. Thus, no ascorbic acid equates to no vitamin C, according to them."

In the same paper cited above, Richard outlines further reasons why synthetic ascorbic acid should be avoided. They include the fact that nearly all synthetic vitamin C supplements today are manufactured from genetically modified (GMO) corn, beets, tapioca, or cassava. In addition, he writes, *"Synthetic ascorbic acid has been shown to destroy beneficial probiotic bacteria in the human gut and to cause oxidative stress...Ascorbic acid supplements can speed up the process of arteriosclerosis...and ascorbic acid can also cause DNA damage."*

While researching the benefits of whole food vitamin C-complex and the detriments of synthetic vitamin C supplements, I came across a study of Iranian Paralympics athletes that examined the vitamin and mineral composition of the athletes' bodies. (Amirsasan R et al, 2017, *Int J Basic Sci Med*;2(3):123-127.) What the researchers discovered was that the athletes' iron levels were approximately ten times greater than any other mineral they were studying, and, of the vitamins, vitamin C was also about ten times greater. The study's findings further confirmed for me that whole food vitamin C-complex is instrumental in managing iron, keeping it from becoming unbound and wreaking havoc in the body, whereas synthetic ascorbic acid/ ascorbate does just the opposite. It allows iron to become unbound and to build up excessively in the body's tissues. It is vitally important that you fully understand that.

It is also important to understand that synthetic ascorbic acid, despite claims to the contrary, is not viewed purely as an antioxidant, but under proper conditions, in the presence of excess iron, is considered a pro-oxidant (Pavlovic et al, 2005, Antioxidant and Pro-Oxidant Effect of Ascorbic Acid. *Acta Medica Medianae* 44(1): 65-68). It is whole food vitamin C-complex that is the more complete antioxidant, meaning that it stops the oxidative (rusting) process that is caused by iron that pervades our body.

Synthetic Vitamin C and Ceruloplasmin: The reason why synthetic vitamin C enables iron to become unbound and excessive, thereby causing oxidative stress, is because of how it interacts with and destroys the master antioxidant protein: ceruloplasmin. This is confirmed by the following facts.

FACT: Ceruloplasmin has that name because this oxidase enzyme presents as the color "sky blue," specifically because of four $Cu(I)$ atoms encircling an oxygen molecule deep inside the proteins structure.

FACT: When ceruloplasmin loses its principal enzyme (ferroxidase) function, it becomes decolorized, otherwise called "bleached."

FACT: Ascorbic acid (synthetic vitamin C) causes ceruloplasmin to lose its color and lose its ferroxidase enzyme function that is essential to regulate and mobilize iron. (Holmberg & Laurell, 1948; Scheinberg & Morrell, 1958; Scheinberg & Sternlieb, 1960; Percival & Harris, 1987; 1988; 1989; 1990; Harris ED 1990.)

To properly understand and interpret the research that addresses the interactions between synthetic ascorbic acid and ceruloplasmin, it is essential that you understand that this is not a typical protein and it does not express just one function. I have identified over 20 enzyme functions for ceruloplasmin, in addition to one of its known roles as a transport protein to restore copper status in tissue throughout our body. Three of those enzyme functions are particularly noteworthy for this discussion. Ceruloplasmin:

- Regulates iron metabolism (ferroxidase enzyme, aka FOX)
- Regulates reactive oxygen species or ROS (SOD, CAT, GPx, PON-1)
- Regulates Nitric Oxide (NO*) via nitrite reductase enzyme.

Our challenge when it comes to making sense of our world is to recognize that we tend to think in a "binary" fashion. We see the world as either this way or that way: left or right; on or off. That is how we have been trained to think. It is very difficult to understand a biological protein—*one of the most important in the human body*—that has eight copper atoms and more than 20 simultaneous enzyme functions. That concept is very hard to fathom, and, I would suggest, nearly impossible for mainstream medicine to accept, let alone incorporate, into their reductionist model of "healthcare." This research model of seeking to isolate ceruloplasmin's transport function is ludicrous, at best. Know that the basis of Big Pharma science is one gene, one protein, one function. Ceruloplasmin, by its design, complexity and functionality, shatters this childlike, reductionist paradigm that undergirds the entire pharmaceutical industry.

There is a rich legacy and trail of research that demonstrates and documents the known properties of ceruloplasmin as a copper transport protein, dating back to at least 1954 (Berne & Kunkel) and continuing well into this century (Baker Z et al. 2017). Despite these well documented findings, doctors are not taught about this fundamental property of ceruloplasmin to transport copper around the body, and are never taught to measure ceruloplasmin levels, nor its enzyme activities, especially its ferroxidase function that is essential for proper iron recycling and iron metabolism activities. Please know that there is a major difference in knowing the "level" of ceruloplasmin protein versus the "activity" of its key enzyme, ferroxidase. It is the difference between knowing the number of cars in a parking lot, and the number of cars on a highway.

There is also a long and rich trail of research documenting the ascorbic acid/ascorbate disruption of copper absorption and function. When addressing the ascorbic acid-ceruloplasmin interaction, we need to also consider the extensive body of research about the known effect of ascorbic acid to inhibit copper absorption in the intestine and/or accelerate its excretion via bile action, along with its known ability to increase iron levels in the liver, beginning with the pioneering research of Hart et al, 1928, regarding copper-iron dynamics. What follows is a list of subsequent studies that have added to our understanding of these dynamics.

1962, Briggs MH, "Possible Relations of Ascorbic Acid, Ceruloplasmin and Toxic Aromatic Metabolites [referring to Adrenochrome…] in Schizophrenia."

1968, Van Campen & Gross, "Influence of Ascorbic Acid on the Absorption of Copper by Rats."

1970, Hunt et al, "Copper Deficiency in Chicks: Effects of Ascorbic Acid on Iron, Copper, Cytochrome Oxidase Activity, and Aortic Mucopolysaccharides." (Key Finding: "Supplementing the Cu[copper]-deficient diet with 0.5% L-ascorbic acid increased mortality 40%, raised total ascorbic acid mucopolysaccharides to a higher level, and increased liver iron by 36%.)

1970, Hunt et al, "Interrelationships between Copper deficiency and Dietary Ascorbic Acid in the Rabbit." (Key Findings: "Signs of Cu deficiency, including reduced growth, achromotrichia and alopecia, anemia, and gross alterations in the bones of the forelimbs, developed most rapidly in those animals fed ascorbic acid; compared with the controls, the concentration of liver cu decreased and that of liver iron increased (>50%) in Cu-deficient animals; and cytochrome oxidase was reduced in liver and heart in cu-deficient animals, this effect was accentuated in heart preparations from animals fed ascorbic acid.")

1971, Hoffer A, "Ascorbic Acid and Toxicity."

1981, Disilvestro & Harris, "A Post-absorption Effect of L-Ascorbic Acid on Copper Metabolism in Chicks." (Key Finding: "The studies confirm the antagonistic properties of L-ascorbic acid on copper metabolism...")

1982, Solomons & Viteri, "Biological Interactions of Ascorbic Acid & Mineral Nutrients" (Key Findings: "In the intestine, ascorbic acid enhances the absorption of dietary iron and selenium; reduces the absorption of copper, nickel, & manganese; but apparently has little effect on zinc or cobalt... At the tissue level, iron overload enhances the oxidative catabolism of ascorbic acid.")

1983, Finley FB et al, "Influence of Ascorbic Acid Supplementation on Copper Status in Young Adult Men." (Key Finding: "Although observed effects occurred within physiological ranges of normal values, this study confirms that a high ascorbic acid intake is antagonistic to copper status of men as has been demonstrated in laboratory animals.")

1987, Jacob RA et al: (Key Finding: "Dietary ascorbate has been found to interfere with copper absorption and in the high AA [ascorbic acid] supplementation group, there is a 21% loss of oxidase activity.")

The above are only a small selection of such studies that confirm the negative impacts that synthetic vitamin C have on our health. In summary, what they document is that ascorbic acid kills ceruloplasmin, and lowers copper absorption in the intestine, while enhancing iron absorption—precisely three outcomes that you DO NOT want to occur if you desire good health and optimal energy production!

Other research that I want to call your attention to was conducted by Drs. Susan S. Percival and Edward D. Harris in the 1980s and 1990s. The focus of these studies was related to the field of oncology and oncologists' obsession with chelating copper from the body. What Percival and Harris did was confirm a mechanism by which ascorbic acid would "liberate" copper from ceruloplasmin and then apply copper chelators to remove that copper from tissue. Among their key findings:

- Data suggested that the ceruloplasmin protein and copper had separated and only the copper had penetrated the K-562 cells.
- Thus, copper transport from ceruloplasmin shows a clear departure from iron transport via transferrin (one of ceruloplasmin's key functions) in these same cells.
- The role of ceruloplasmin – in transport – ends at the cell surface.

Hopefully, the information above provides you with a more complete picture of the known and studied interactions between synthetic vitamin C (ascorbic acid), copper, and ceruloplasmin. It is by no means exhaustive, but it offers an overview of the key metabolic challenges that ascorbic acid brings to copper metabolism, and most especially ceruloplasmin, the key copper protein that serves innumerable antioxidant roles in the human metabolism. *It explains why synthetic ascorbic acid is one of the most important STOPS in the Root Cause Protocol, and why whole food vitamin C-complex is most important STARTS of the RCP.*

In Chapter 7, I stated that whole food vitamin C-complex is analogous to an entire car, complete with the steering wheel, the engine, the tires, and a shell (exterior cover), whereas synthetic ascorbic acid by itself is just the car's outer shell. Period. When it comes to the vitamin C-complex and your health, you want to be sure that you are getting the entire "automobile." You can only do so by supplementing with whole food vitamin C-complex. So, when choosing a vitamin C supplement, get in the habit of reading the ingredients label. If it lists ascorbic acid or ascorbate, please put it down and look for a product with a label that says whole food vitamin C and lists food sources such as camu camu, rose hips, berry extracts, acerola cherry extract, cranberry, and/or other food sources of the entire vitamin C-complex. You and your copper-dependent metabolites will thank you for this discernment and this extra effort.

D-etonating the Vitamin D Myth

"People would rather believe the simple lie, than the complex truth."

~ Alexis de Tocqueville (1805 – 1859)

To begin this discussion about vitamin D, let me take you back to the 1950s, when another nutritional myth began that led to dire consequences in our nation's health. I am referring, of course, to the Cholesterol Myth, which began in earnest following President

Dwight D. Eisenhower's initial heart attack (Sept 24, 1955). Once that occurred, the world was taken hostage and put on a low-fat diet. The expressed target of that dietary regimen was to lower our intake of cholesterol that was being identified as the "cause" of the alarming rise of heart disease and cardiac deaths following World War II. What was NOT expressed was the fact that these regressive dietary recommendations led to a significant reduction of retinol (real vitamin-A) from the SAD, American/Western world diet, which had a devastating effect on copper physiology, which resulted in a devastating effect on human health. This was entirely due to misleading and myth-leading clinical studies based solely on *correlation*, and not *causation*.

It was not until Ravsnkov, Diamond et al, 2016, published their definitive study that this global deception ended once and for all. In fact, it is not cholesterol that causes heart disease, but the lipid peroxidation ("rusting") of cholesterol, which is caused entirely by increased dietary iron in the grains due to iron fortification programs that began in 1941 in the UK, Canada, and the United States. In the US, there was a 50 percent increase in iron being added as of 1969. In addition, the rise of added sugars and omega-6 oils added insult to injury of iron fortification. Sixty-five years of circular, clinical insanity was brought to a much needed close by that critical and definitive study in 2016.

What we are now witnessing is the "Son Of Cholesterol Myth," with the equally mind-numbing distortion of truth with the "D"iatribes and "D"eception around "vitamin-D deficiency." Please know that it is entirely a fabricated condition, relying on flawed metrics that are based on the difference between a "fuel gauge" (purely a high/low function) versus miles per gallon that involves multiple variables. What follows will bring important facts to light to explain just how wrong, and just how toxic, this dietary recommendation is.

The first thing you must understand about vitamin D, as I pointed out in Chapter 7, is that it is NOT a vitamin at all. In reality, it is technically a secosteroid hormone, which is why I refer to it as hormone D. I'm passionately opposed to vitamin D-only supplementation because MTHR Nature never-intended that we would supplement with it as a synthetic "nutrient." And, until the last 20 years or so, we didn't. Then everything changed, largely due to the efforts of one man, Michael F. Holick, PhD, MD, a Boston University endocrinologist. His promotion of supplemental D, in tandem with the Vitamin D Council and the Endocrine Society, resulted in what the *New York Times* described as an annual "billion-dollar vitamin D sales and testing juggernaut" due to Holick's published papers and his book, *The Vitamin D Solution*, that warned of widespread vitamin D deficiencies throughout America, and which called for a massive expansion of testing of vitamin D levels.

In addition, Holick's misguided recommendations led doctors to believe that healthy vitamin D levels needed to be at least 30 nanograms per milliliter, and ideally between 50 to 70 ng/mL and even higher, whereas, previously, levels at or slightly above 20 ng/mL were considered sufficient. This lower level, as you learned in Chapter 8, was precisely what Dr. Mohammed Amer, MD, and his colleagues at Johns Hopkins University showed in 2013 was all that is required for optimal health.

Today, however, Dr. Amer's findings are ignored and physicians and commercial diagnostic labs have universally adopted Holick's much higher levels as their standard. Much to the detriment of their patients' and clients' health, but to the financial benefit of Holick and other physicians, organizations, labs, and vitamin supplement companies who continue to push the vitamin D myth. (Szabo, Liz. Vitamin D, the Sunshine Supplement, Has Shadowy Money Behind It. *New York Times*. Aug 18, 2018.) As Dr. Amer points out, "Healthy people have been popping these pills, but they should not continue taking vitamin D supplements unchecked. At a certain point, more vitamin D no longer confers any survival benefit, so taking these expensive supplements is at best a waste of money." At worst, doing so might accelerate our "D"emise.

That is not hyperbole on my part. It is a fact that was documented in a scientific paper published in *The American Journal of Medicine* in 2015 which found that blood levels of vitamin D between 50 and 75 ng/mL (considered to be optimal by Holick, etc.) can increase the risk of all-cause mortality, as well as the risk for heart disease and various types of cancer. (Taylor CL et al, 2015-Nov 1, Questions About Vitamin D for Primary Care Practice. *Amer J Med*;128(11):1167-1170).

Another important vitamin D researcher is Meg Mangin, RN, cofounder of Chronic Illness Recovery, a free counseling service for physicians, nurses, and patients, exploring inflammation therapy (for more information, see www.ci-recovery.org). Among her many noteworthy accomplishments, Mangin served on a National Institutes of Health (NIH) State of the Science panel, and served on an NIH Data, Safety and Monitoring Board for six years. She is also the co-author of a very important research paper on vitamin D that was published in the science journal *Inflammation Research* in 2014 (Mangin M, Sinha R, Fincher K, 2014-Jul 22, Inflammation and vitamin D: the infection connection, *Inflamm Res*;63(10):803-19).

The essential thesis of that paper, which Mangin and her co-authors thoroughly support with other published studies, is that low blood levels of storage D (25 dihydroxy vitamin D, or 25 (OH) D, the type that is tested for) are found in both healthy and sick people. This calls into question the necessity for vitamin D testing. Just as importantly, she notes, *"The current method of determining vitamin D status may be at fault. The level of 25(OH)D does not always reflect the level of 1,25-dihydroxyvitamin-D (1,25(OH)2D)."* Please do

NOT confuse the actions of Storage-D and Active-D. *They are NOT interchangeable and they are NOT synonymous with each other.*

As we learned in Chapter 7, active Hormone-D, 1,25-dihydroxyvitamin-D3, is the bioactive form of vitamin D which does all the heavy lifting in your body's immune system when complexed with the vitamin-D receptor (VDR) and a KEY nuclear receptor, RXR. Working together, that triad is noteworthy. It is important to note, however, that RXR is a metabolite from vitamin A and high doses of supplemental D block vitamin A's absorption and thus its many functions in the body. (Please re-read that sentence, again, to grasp its full meaning.)

In addition, Mangin's research paper pointed out that, although vitamin D is commonly recommended to prevent and reverse chronic inflammation, studies do not demonstrate that vitamin D does this. In fact, the evidence suggests just the opposite. *Low storage D status is solely an indication that there is inflammation in the body due solely to high unbound iron and low magnesium.* You can ingest buckets of supplemental D and NEVER correct the underlying inflammation caused by the mineral dynamics of excess iron in the tissues and subsequent loss of magnesium inside the cell.

In *Supplementing For Low Vitamin D? Not So Fast*, an article written for laypeople to explain her research findings, Mangin explains what happens when vitamin D is produced in the skin due to sunlight exposure. *"This molecule is transported to the liver where it is used to produce calcidiol [storage D]. This storage form of vitamin D [25(OH)D] is transported to the kidneys where it is converted to the active form of vitamin D, called calcitriol [1,25 dihydroxyvitamin-D]."*

Then she adds this kicker: "In sick people, low calcidiol (often labeled as vitamin D deficiency) and high calcitriol are markers of a chronic inflammatory process. Low calcidiol is a consequence of a disease process, not a cause. *Supplementing with vitamin D increases the level of calcidiol, making it easier for the body to produce excess calcitriol, which increases inflammatory symptoms* (emphasis added).

"Numerous studies have shown that people living in very sunny countries have levels of calcidiol that are being labeled as vitamin D deficient despite the fact that these people are healthy. *This suggests that 'low' calcidiol is normal in healthy individuals.* (emphasis added) *Studies of disease occurrence have not shown that taking vitamin D supplements to increase calcidiol has a beneficial effect.*" (https:// fearlessparent.org/supplementing-low-vitamin-d-not-so-fast)

The crux of Mangin's research is that low storage vitamin D is simply a sign of a *consequence* of high inflammation, *it is not the cause.* We can take supplemental D all day long, but we're not going to change the level of cellular inflammatory state.

Why?

Because we're not going to be restoring magnesium by taking vitamin D, and we're not going to correct the problem with iron by taking vitamin D. In fact, I would argue we're only going to make these problems worse.

One of the other important conclusions from her research is that people who are healthy have low levels of storage vitamin D and what's deemed normal levels of active D. Conversely, people who are considered sick or chronically ill also have low storage D, but they also have elevated levels of active D. Their bodies are using that active D, which is being produced outside of the kidney tissue and is known as extra renal bioactive vitamin D, as an antimicrobial peptide (AMP) to try to kill the pathogens that are living on the excess iron that is in the body because the storage vitamin D is shutting down vitamin A metabolism, and it's not allowing the proper recycling of iron.

All of these interactions are connected. Given the stress levels on this planet, there's not enough magnesium in the body, and there's too much iron. Inflammation itself is not a disease. Rather, it's a clear indication of metabolic imbalance caused by this mineral dysregulation, which, in this case, is initiated and then perpetuated by taking vitamin D supplements. The leading research is clearly demonstrating that low vitamin D, or low storage D, is a clinical sign of inflammation. The continued misguided recommendations by doctors to "take more supplemental D" is another example supporting my premise that we've been misled and misfed.

Let's go back in time and dig even deeper. In 1982, William Weglicki and his colleague, Terry Phillips, published breakthrough research clearly establishing that magnesium deficiency is the cellular mineral state that precedes the inflammatory cascade in the body. Then we find that the flip side is also true: Less calcium, especially in a magnesium deficient state, is protective against inflammation. The reason why is because it is magnesium that regulates calcium in the body, just as copper regulates iron. These are the metabolic roles that these minerals are intended to play in the body These are all scientifically verified facts, yet they are not widely known.

Too much calcium in the body is going to drive inflammation. Why? Because excess calcium drives magnesium down and lowers the body's ability to absorb magnesium. That's a very important premise to understand.

What is also vital to understand is that the key to improving hormone D status is, in fact, focusing on magnesium status. This fact was made clear by research conducted by Dr. Xinging Deng, PhD, in 2013 ("Magnesium, vitamin D status and mortality: results from US NHANES 2001-2006 and NHANES III.") What Dr. Deng examined was magnesium and vitamin D status in relation to overall mortality from the National Health and Nutrition Examination Survey (NHANES) data compiled from 2001 to 2006. The findings are very clear, and show that magnesium intake alone or its interaction with vitamin D intake influences vitamin D status.

As Deng's study documented, magnesium is required in order to metabolize, transport and regulate hormone D. There are no less than eight enzymes in hormone D metabolism that require magnesium. The protein that transports the precursor to vitamin D to the liver requires magnesium, as well. In addition, the 25-hydroxylase enzyme inside the liver must have magnesium as its catalyst, and the circulating vitamin D-binding protein also needs to have magnesium.

It is also very important to understand is that both vitamin A and D must be taken together because they are biological partners. It's not a question of vitamin A versus D, it's a question of A and D working together. There's a reason why they're found together in nature, especially in nutrient-rich cod liver oil. Mother Nature knows why they need to be together much better than physicians and Big Pharma do, I would contend.

As you learned earlier in this book, retinol (real vitamin A) is essential for the body's production of iron regulatory proteins and, especially, ceruloplasmin. That's a *big* deal. High supplemental D intake causes low vitamin A absorption. Both substances share the same receptor sites in the body, and if vitamin D starts flooding into the body, vitamin A cannot be absorbed and is compromised. When retinol is compromised, iron becomes dysregulated, causing it to be to be found with increased frequency inside the cell and its storage protein, ferritin, to increase inside the blood, which is an important inflammatory marker.

We've being trained, like circus bears, to believe that we need only supplemental D to solve this problem of chronic inflammation, when, for a fact, the body is elegantly designed to use magnesium to correct both low storage hormone D and the inflammation associated with low magnesium, high calcium, and excess, unbound iron. Resolving chronic inflammation has never been a storage (supplemental) D issue. That's where mainstream medicine has it completely wrong. Few doctors understand the physiology of what is driving the synthesis and the activation of storage hormone D and what hormone D's relationship is with retinol. This vital understanding is completely lost on doctors and other health practitioners all across the globe.

Another thing that is often ignored by physicians is what happens when hormone D is produced in the body. Typically, this process is summarized by saying when it is obtained via sunlight or diet, storage D is synthesized first in the liver, and then activated in the kidneys. But as I wrote above, it can also be activated outside of the kidneys in a process known as extra renal activation. Moreover, once activated in the kidneys, hormone D can go one of ten different ways. It's commonly assumed that D only automatically goes from a storage state to a bioactive state, but there are other states it can convert to, as well, depending on what our bodies need. This is rarely addressed by physicians and other hormone D proponents. All of their testing is based upon the storage level, with no testing for these other metabolic outcomes. I think that's a very significant omission that results in a lot of needless confusion and needs to be considered when assessing a person's hormone D status. Measuring levels of storage D is not enough; to be fully responsible and responsive, both of hormone D's key metabolites (storage and active) must also be assessed.

This ties back into the findings of Mohammed Amer, MD, and his colleagues that showed there is no clinical benefit to having storage D levels above 21 ng/mL. Dr. Amer was examining the data sets for both all-cause mortality and cardiovascular disease mortality, and what he found isn't what mainstream medicine wants you to believe. He drew some very important conclusions from this particular study, the clinical significance of which is that there's an inverse association between storage D and all cause and cardiovascular disease mortality. In healthy adults, there seems to be no additional protection by having storage D levels above 21 ng/mL.

What Dr. Amer and his colleagues are suggesting is that the entire hormone D reference range should be rethought. A somewhat heretical idea, as you can well imagine, since today optimum levels of storage D are claimed to be at least 50 ng/mL and above. This means that nearly all of the people who are deemed to be deficient in storage D actually are not. It's a false flag marker, because the starting point is set well above the conclusions of Dr. Amer's very important study. I think its conclusions are very sound, however controversial they might appear in the face of what most physicians believe and advocate about currently promoted hormone D levels. His findings reveal some very important concepts that challenge some of the current hormone D mythology.

As you read this, you might be wondering, *But what about all the claims that vitamin D protects against cancer?*

That's a very good question, considering how frequently these claims are bandied about. The answer, once again, is that these claims are also more myth than fact. Proof of this can be found in two studies that were done a decade apart by Dr. Joan Lappe, at Tufts University, School of Nutrition.

In 2007, Dr. Lappe and her colleagues conducted a randomized clinical trial that examined vitamin D and calcium supplementation as potential anticancer agents for postmenopausal women. Their conclusion was that improving calcium and vitamin D nutritional status substantially reduced all cancer risk in postmenopausal women. This study, along with others like it, influenced the thinking of many physicians, oncologists, internists, and OB-GYN practitioners and led to the status vitamin D continues to have as a cancer protector.

However, in 2017, Dr. Lappe oversaw a follow-up study (Lappe JM et al, 2017, "Effect of Vitamin D and Calcium Supplementation on Cancer Incidence in Older Women" https://jamanetwork.com/journals/jama/fullarticle/2613159). Once again, they examined healthy postmenopausal women with the same mean baseline sample of storage D levels (32.8 ng/mL) who supplemented with vitamin D and calcium, and compared them with a placebo group. This time, Lappe and her colleagues found that supplementing with vitamin D and calcium did not result in a significantly lower risk of all cancer types at four years out, compared to the placebo group. This was a stunning reversal of their previous study that ballyhooed the idea that more vitamin D would help correct cancer. They re-studied it and they retracted their position!

Yet, to this day, most physicians still continue to tell their patients they had better supplement with vitamin D to prevent cancer despite the fact that we now know that vitamin D supplementation does not offer the anticancer protection that most people think it does. It is very important to challenge this mindless assertion that we need more vitamin D. We don't. We need more magnesium and bioavailable copper.

Another important factor to understand when considering vitamin D is that there is a major difference between supplemental D coming out of a vitamin bottle versus vitamin D that comes via the transactions triggered by sunlight. Vitamin D produced by sunlight exposure is sulfated, meaning that it is water-soluble. It has completely different properties than supplemental D, which are fat-soluble. As Stephanie Seneff, PhD notes, vitamin D must be sulfated to have access to cells all over the body. Fat-soluble vitamin D is incapable of circulating through the body in the same way that the sun-derived natural, sulfated form of vitamin D does. Instead, when we consume vitamin D as a supplement, we store it. This fact has been established by the pioneering work of Dr. Stephanie Seneff. As she and her colleagues showed, taking synthetic supplemental D ignores the natural function of converting sun-kissed 7-dehydrocholesterol into the precursor to vitamin D. By ingesting supernatural doses of synthetic supplemental D, the body is being robbed of its natural mechanism to keep cholesterol levels in proper regulation. What this also does is prevent the production of sulfated vitamin D, the water-soluble form that the body seeks to have access to for healthy functions. (De Luca 1997; Seneff S, 2010 www.sciencedirect.com/topics/neuroscience/7-dehydrochloresterol; https://people.csail.mit.edu/seneff/sulfur_obesity_alzheimers_muscle_wasting.html)

Could the massive consumption of vitamin D supplements over the past two decades be a hidden factor further contributing to obesity, heart disease, and chronic fatigue?

When the ultraviolet (UV) photons of sunlight touch our skin they interact with cholesterol chemicals in the skin, providing energy that "excites" the chemicals, causing them to break up so that they become the precursor to vitamin D, as well as producing an abundance of cholesterol sulfate. In Dr. Seneff's opinion, this is the more important molecule, and I absolutely agree with her. Many of the alleged benefits of hormone D are actually the benefits of cholesterol sulfate. The protection against cancer, diabetes, and cardiovascular disease, and the improved immune function that modern medicine attributes to storage D is really due to this sulfated form of cholesterol, as opposed the supplemental form of vitamin D.

All of the benefits ascribed to vitamin D are also actually a direct function of the active-D metabolite and not the storage form that is always measured. There is no responsible measurement of active hormone-D. This is patently absurd! This metabolite is a hormone, and whenever doctors measure hormones, they always seek to know their storage levels and active status. Furthermore, there is a key ratio of active-to-storage D status. According to Kenny De Meirleir, MD, PhD, a world-renowned endocrinologist in the Netherlands, the value of active D should never exceed 1.5 to 2.0 times the level of storage D. When it does, this is a sign of an infection and indicates that active-D is being turned into AMP (Acute Microbial Peptides) to fight the pathogens, all of which are living on excess, unbound iron.

When I first became aware of this process of sunlight converting cholesterol chemicals into vitamin D, I wanted to understand more about the physics of light. It's an absolutely fascinating subject. The key is that light has a frequency and that frequency is 126 hertz (Hz). This frequency is measured as a wavelength in nanometers, and it's 560 nanometers, which is the exact same wavelength of green light. Even though the sun appears yellow, it's emitting the frequency of green light, which is why plants that are green relate to the sun. Green wavelengths of light are critical for photosynthesis. Please know, even more demanding and dynamic than copper <> iron metabolism is the physics of light. It is extraordinary!

I was really intrigued when I stumbled upon that because it's not what we would intuitively think. Proponents of color therapy, a healing modality that uses light to improve health, have long pointed out that the green wavelength of light is the one that is most effective for supporting health at its most basic, foundational level. Yet, for decades, we've all been advised to limit our exposure to sunlight because it causes skin cancer, especially if you have very fair skin.

Well, what does very fair skin mean? It means you don't have enough bioavailable copper, and retinol to activate the tyrosinase enzyme to make melanin. That's what fair skin is.

So what do we do? We slather all sorts of skin lotion that blocks sunlight and the inflammation that we call sunburn. I grew up with this and know exactly what this is all about. I used to bathe in the lotions. I was terrified of sunlight because it was inevitably very painful. Now I know differently. So let's be very careful about the mainstream message, which is: "Get out of the sun, it's going to kill you". No, we absolutely need the sun. We can't make healthy vitamin D without it.

Sunlight also helps the body to break down vitamin A. Nobody talks about the fact that we have got to breakdown vitamin A in order to make it work. If we can't take retinol and break it into its component parts of retinoic acids and the nuclear receptors RARs, RORs, RXRs, and the RZR receptors we've got metabolic problems on our hands. Sunlight is what makes this vital production of retinoids possible, through a process known technically as "photodegradation," in addition to sunlight triggering the "photosynthesis" of vitamin D. We can't live without either one. Sunshine is the key to both of these "vital amines," as they were called back in the early 20th century.

Now here's another very interesting fact that modern medicine seems to overlook: Copper is essential for these amines, and also greatly benefits from sunlight. Noted researcher Ray Peat, PhD, explained why when he stated, "Sunlight is what keeps copper from becoming iron." Here's how that works. In addition to synthesizing vitamin D and cholesterol sulfates, sunlight is necessary for breaking down retinol into its component parts and allowing retinoic acid to be used inside the cell nucleus. Without enough sunlight, this doesn't happen as efficiently.

In addition, we can't make bioavailable copper without retinol, and copper cannot get loaded into the ceruloplasmin protein without retinol in the diet. Assuming there is enough retinol in the diet, sunlight enhances these processes.

A 2008 study (Mawson AR et al, 2013, "Role of Fat-Soluble Vitamins A and D in the Pathogenesis of Influenza: A New Perspective" www.hindawi.com/journals/isrn/2013/246737/) explains the two sides of this dynamic of both vitamin A and vitamin D metabolism. Modern medicine and everyone else need to stop thinking that it's just vitamin D that we have to be concerned about. Vitamin A and its hormonal metabolites need to be considered, as well, along with the essential need to increase the bioavailability of copper.

All of this is accomplished through the metabolic pathways that depend on the natural stimulation of various receptor sites in the body. For example, if we don't have enough retinol (vitamin A) in our diet, we can't activate the receptor sites for vitamin D, known as VDR. The recognized actions of active D are dependent on the action of these vitamin D receptors, which, in turn, are dependent on the RXR nuclear receptors that are only available when retinol, real vitamin A, is in the diet (von Essen et al, 2018, "VDR: The Vitamin D Receptor." *Encyclopedia of Signaling Molecules*).

As I stated in Chapter 7, in order to have its fullest expression, vitamin D needs to be complexed with RXR, which requires retinol, as well, because RXR is a retinoid receptor. I'm not trying to turn you into a geneticist, but I want you to understand that this metabolite that you've probably never heard of is instrumental in the function of vitamin D working in your body. It is the master regulatory nuclear receptor in the body and is linked to over a dozen different nuclear receptors. This is why vitamin A is so vital to your health. Without enough of it, your body cannot perform as our Maker and MTHR Nature intended. Given the lack of vitamin A in the typical American diet dating back to 1955, this might be part of the reason why we have so many genetic defects occurring today.

All of the fame and glory attributed to hormone D is really due to the combined ability of VDR and RXR as they form a protein complex called a heterodimer that then engages the necessary gene transcription actions to affect the immune system. This necessary step is entirely ignored in mainstream medicine. Truth be known, RXR is one of the most important nuclear regulatory ligands in our metabolism that is lost to people still following low-fat diets. This nutrient is one of the "hidden hungers" that is causing the endless metabolic dysfunctions that undermine and destroy our health.

You also need to understand that hormone D's active metabolites show up in monocytes, dendritic cells, memory T cells, and B cells, all of which are key cells in our body's immune system. Hormone D taken as a supplement does not always become the storage and then active forms of hormone D. In fact, synthetic vitamin D can go in 12 different directions, because there are 12 different metabolites that can be formed depending on the internal requirements of the individual taking this supplement(s). They all have a need for vitamin D receptors (VDR), which means that they also all have a need for RXR. They cannot work without that. Your immune system needs both sides of these nutritional components. Without both, your body can't recreate and translate the genetic code properly. That fact seems to be lost on mainstream nutrition.

What also seems to be lost is the fact that supplemental D shuts down that entire process. Supplemental D prevents the absorption of retinol, and the higher the dose of D you take, the less retinol that will be available you, resulting in a wide range of health problems. The very same problems that Supplemental D is claimed to prevent and resolve. (Mawson AR et al, 2013, Role of Fat-Soluble Vitamins A and D in the Pathogenesis of Influenza: A New Perspective. *Int Scholarly Res Notices.* July 19. 2012; Volume 2013 |Article ID 246737.)

In addition, contrary to another popular opinion associated with the hormone D myth, there is no relationship between the active D [1,25(OH)2D3] status and the hormone D metabolite that is essential for building bone matrix, 24r, 25-dihydroxyvitamin D. This critical metabolite needed for bone integrity is actually more related to the status of parathyroid hormone, and not active-D. And parathyroid hormone, like all of the calcium-regulating hormones, depends on magnesium status. (Bosworth et al, 2012, The serum 24r,25 dihydroxyvitamin D concentration, a Marker of Vitamin D Catabolism, is Reduced in CKD. *Kidney Inst.* Sept; 82(6): 693-700.)

Moreover, a series of studies conducted by researchers at the University of Auckland, Australia, conclusively demonstrated that hormone D supplements not only do not improve bone integrity, they also increase calcification of tissue.

(Falls, 2014: https://pubmed.ncbi.nlm.nih.gov/24768505/;

Bone, 2014: https://pubmed.ncbi.nlm.nih.gov/24703049/)

The following studies provide further examples of the known, health-damaging metabolic/mineral impacts that hormone D supplements cause:

Renal Potassium Wasting: Ferris et al, 1962, "Renal Potassium-Wasting Induced by Vitamin D" https://pubmed.ncbi.nlm.nih.gov/13892592/

Loss of Renal Energy Production and Increased Iron Storage: Zager et al, 1999, "Calcitriol Directly Sensitizes Renal Tubular Cells to ATP-Depletion- and Iron-mediated

Attack" https://www.ncbi.nlm.nih.gov/pmc/articles/PMC1866639/

1,25-dihydroxyvitamin D3 increases synthesis of metallothionein that binds up copper: Karasawa et al, 1987, "Regulation of metallothionein gene expression by 1 alpha,25dihydroxyvitamin D3 in cultured cells and in mice" https://www.ncbi.nlm.nih.gov/pmc/articles/PMC299640/

Vitamin D suppresses hepcidin and ferritin synthesis which causes increased iron storage in the cell: Barcchetta et al, 2014, "Suppression of Iron-Regulatory Hepcidin by Vitamin D" https://www.ncbi.nlm.nih.gov/pmc/articles/PMC3935584/

Increased cellular iron lowers pH and oxygen: Wilson DF et al, 2012, "Oxygen, pH, and Mitochondrial Oxidative Phosphorylation" https://pubmed.ncbi.nlm.nih.gov/23104697/.

Having comprehended all of the above, I think you get the point. There is not one shred of evidence that supplemental hormone D, acting alone or in isolation of vitamin A, confers any benefit of any kind. So, please don't be taken in by the oft-repeated calls by physicians to increase your intake of supplemental D. Such recommendations are madness, and will only "D"iminish your health!

Other Elements of the RCP–The Non-Nutritional "X-Factors" (Phase X)

"Good, better, best. Never let it rest. 'Til your good is better and your better is best."

– St. Jerome (347–419/420)

"In the process of letting go, you will lose many things from the past, but you will find yourself."

– Deepak Chopra, MD

While following the STOPS and the STARTS of the three Phases of the RCP that you learned about in chapters 7 and 8 are the most essential steps you must take to banish fatigue and protect yourself from "metabolic dysfunction," commonly known as "medical disease," the following additional, non-nutritional recommendations, which we call the "X-Factors," should also be considered. In my experience, after over a decade consulting with others and helping them progress on the RCP, each of the factors below can significantly enhance all of the health benefits the RCP provides, including hastening how quickly you experience them. Each of these X-Factors can be implemented at any time.

These first four factors are most important to address as any one of them, or a combination of them, can block the intended impact of the RCP nutrients.

1) START Clearing Food And Environmental Allergies and Sensitivities

Food allergies and sensitivities are among the most commonly misdiagnosed undiagnosed medical conditions in the US. An estimated 10 to 30 percent of the population suffers from this form of environmentally triggered illness, and approximately 95 percent of them have not been properly identified and treated.

Though the concept of food allergies remains controversial among conventional physicians, it is not new. Hippocrates, for instance, discovered that milk could trigger hives and gastrointestinal upset in certain people. Despite the fact that food allergies are becoming increasingly common, they remain one of the most misdiagnosed conditions.

Ironically, people who suffer from food allergies often crave the very foods that are harmful for them. People who are allergic to wheat, for example, will often have pasta or bread throughout the week and feel deprived if they don't. Common food allergens include milk and dairy products, wheat, corn, tomato products, peanuts, chocolates, and shellfish, as well as food additives, dyes, and preservatives. Virtually any food or beverage can cause allergic reactions in susceptible people, however.

Numerous substances in the environment, including inside your home, can also cause chronic allergic and sensitivity reactions. These include the pesticides, herbicides, and the nearly 100,000 kinds of other chemicals used by various industries today, less than five percent of which have ever been tested for their effects on human health. Toxic molds and volatile organic compounds (VOCs) in homes and in the workplace can also cause a wide range of severe health problems, as can the many pollutants in the air and drinking water, depending on where you live. Telltale signs of food and/or environmental allergies and sensitivities include:

- Dark circles, swelling, or wrinkles under the eyes
- Runny or stuffy nose
- Postnasal drip
- Excessive mucus
- Watery eyes and/or blurred vision
- Ringing of the ears
- Recurrent ear infections
- Sinusitis
- Sore throats, hoarseness, or chronic coughing
- Coated tongue
- Chest congestion
- Heart palpitations
- Vascular headaches
- Gagging
- Mucus or undigested food in the stool
- Nausea
- Vomiting
- Diarrhea and/or constipation
- Bloating after meals
- Flatulence
- Abdominal pains or cramping
- Extreme thirst
- Hives or rashes
- Dermatitis
- Brittle nails and hair

- Dry skin
- Dandruff
- Skin pallor
- Joint pain
- Frequent or urgent urination
- PMS
- Unnatural or persistent fatigue or drowsiness, anxiety, depression, or panic attacks
- Irritability
- Mental dullness, concentration problems, or confusion
- Faintness or dizziness
- Sleepiness soon after a meal, insomnia or restless sleep

If you or your loved ones suffer from any of the above symptoms, then some form of food allergy may be to blame, especially if symptoms are chronic and do not respond to medical treatments.

Fortunately, there are effective alternatives to such treatments. The two that I most often recommend are NAET and Advanced Allergy Therapeutics (known as AAT in the US and HWA in Australia).

NAET: NAET stands for Nambudripad Allergy Elimination Technique, and is named after its developer, Devi S. Nambudripad, DC, LAc, MD, PhD (Acu). According to Dr. Nambudripad, NAET not only makes it easier to determine the various allergens that may be playing a hidden role in disease, it also allows patients to continue to use or be exposed to the implicated substances without further suffering.

The key to how NAET works lies in its ability to retrain the patient's brain and nervous system to no longer react to the substances s/he is allergic to. This is a radically different approach than the more common method of avoiding allergy triggers for an extended period of time or even a lifetime, once they've been detected.

Part of NAET's success also lies with the body's energy pathways, or meridians, as they are known by acupuncturists. According to Dr.

Nambudripad, when we are exposed to a substance we are allergic or sensitive to our brain and meridian system interprets the substance as being harmful to us. For other people, the substance may be harmless, but for your system it's toxic. As a result, our nervous system "freezes up" in order to defend against it. This, in turn, creates blockages in the meridians. So long as the allergy remains, over time, the blockages lead to further imbalances in the way your body functions.

Allergies themselves, according to Nambudripad, are a response of the immune system to foreign substances around us, or their energy fields. This response triggers different reactions at different times. It depends upon which area of the body is the one where the energy is blocked. The offending substance creates a disturbance in the body's meridian system and that blocks the body's flow of energy, creating imbalance. Reversing that process is what NAET practitioners do. But first they have to know what substances each person is allergic to. They accomplish this through the use of Applied Kinesiology, an offshoot of chiropractic developed by George Goodheart, DC. Patients hold the suspected allergenic substance while the practitioner tests the strength of certain muscles. If an allergy exists, the muscles will exhibit weakness that improves once the patient is no longer in contact with the offending substance.

Once the allergens have been determined, the next step in NAET is to "reprogram" the patient's nervous system to not react to them. This is accomplished by having the patients continue to hold the substance they are allergic to while the NAET practitioner treats them with acupuncture or acupressure. This reprograms the patients' nervous systems to no longer react to the substances they were previously allergic to. As the patients' energy pathways are unblocked while they are holding the substance during the acupuncture treatment, their body stops reacting to it. This, in turn, causes their brains to stop viewing and reacting to the substance as harmful.

Once the treatment is complete, patients are then instructed to avoid exposure to the substance for 25 to 30 hours, after which time they should no longer cause an allergic reaction.

To locate a trained NAET practitioner, please visit www.naet.com

Advanced Allergy Therapeutics (AAT): Like NAET, AAT is based, in part, on some of the principles of acupuncture, as well as chiropractic. Unlike NAET, however, AAT practitioners do not screen for or diagnose allergies and also do not treat the immune system. AAT practitioners view a true allergic reaction as an immune response to an offending substance, which may or may not be harmless to others. By contrast, sensitivities, which account for 98 percent of all cases considered to be allergies, do not impact the immune system. Rather, they cause overreactions in the organs of various other body systems, especially the digestive, respiratory, and dermatological (skin) systems. Instead of focusing on treating sensitivities, the AAT system simply assesses what may be causing a stress to the body and then corrects that stress response.

A further explanation of how AAT works is provided on its website: "Advanced Allergy Therapeutics works directly with the relationship between the major organ systems and inappropriate reactions to harmless substances. While the immune system is responsible for initiating an immune reaction in the case of true allergies, it is the health and state of the organ systems that often determines the type of symptoms that may arise. With both sensitivities and allergies, symptoms typically stem from the organ system affected. For example, one patient may have a reaction to soybean by getting rashes while another patient may react with sinus congestion, heartburn or irritable bowel syndrome. The symptoms in each of these cases represent a different organ system involved. By treating the organ system(s) involved in a reaction, the body is able to respond more appropriately.

"Either the organ system itself may react, causing symptoms, or mast cells located in the tissues may contribute to a reaction. In fact, increasingly, evidence is showing that mast cells, which play a central role in the allergic response, can actually be activated by non-allergic triggers, including stress. This means that the body can exhibit very similar symptoms as those caused by a true allergy, but with no immune involvement at all. However, even in the case of a true allergy, when the reactive organs are treated, the associated symptoms may be reduced or resolved."

According to acupuncture theory, stimulating specific areas (acupoints) on the body, which directly correspond to a specific organ system, improves the health and functioning of that system. The acupoints stimulated during AAT treatments are located along the spine and correspond with the organ systems AAT focus on. "By treating reactive organ systems via these points in relation to an offending substance," the ATT explains, "a defensive state may be altered, allowing for a healthier response. The AAT method does not use needles, but instead utilizes a precision-based acupressure technique to treat the organ systems. This unique approach of addressing defensive physiology is highly effective in altering the state of the organ systems."

To find out more about AAT and to locate an AAT practitioner near you in the United States, please visit www.allergytx.com/home. html. If you live in Australia, please visit www.naturalallergytreatment. com.au which is run by Health & Wellness Australia and Auckland, based in North Sydney, Australia.

2) START Emotional Freedom Technique (EFT)

As we learned previously, stress begins when we feel "out of control," which is how we feel when we have a chronic condition that does NOT respond to stimulus, medications or our endless mental pleadings for it to go away.

Unresolved emotions and stress trigger the creation of fears (I spell it differently: Fe-ar, so we see the symbol for iron), which create a relentless MBR, "magnesium burn rate." (The body loses magnesium in response to any stressor, especially feelings of anxiety or Fe-ar, however subtle or subconscious they may be.)

Sometimes it is necessary to go deeper in order to truly conquer stress because many times the cause of the stress and negative thoughts and emotions we experience are not based in the present, but are being triggered by the effects of past events and the unhealed emotions and beliefs we formed about them. Scientists over the past few decades have discovered that these events and their effects are literally stored within our cells as cellular memories.

Just as your brain records what happens to you each moment, so too do the cells of our body absorb the effects of everything we experience, as well as the interpretations we make of each experience when it occurs. Everything that we have ever perceived, learned, done, and otherwise experienced, and how we interpreted each experience goes into the hopper of our cellular memory to begin generating internal chemical reactions that, unless the cellular memories are healed, can recur for the rest of our life at any time that the cellular memories are triggered. Usually, this triggering process occurs automatically and we aren't even conscious of it happening. Whatever was in your past that lies buried and unhealed within us continues to negatively affect us today and will not stop doing so until our cellular memories of those past events are healed. Quite literally, our issues are in our tissues.

Let me explain further. When we experience "Fe-AR," our tissues contract and our pH becomes acidic. Any farmer will tell you, "acidic soil attracts iron." That's the first half of the cycle: Fe-AR attracts iron. The back half of the cycle, however, is that iron activates the "danger sensor" of the cell, aka NLRP3, which is also called the inflammasome, the nuclear origin of inflammation (Nakamura et al, 2016). Therefore, "Fe-AR ATTRACTS iron and iron ACTIVATES

Fe-AR!" This is an important cornerstone in understanding the mineral/metabolic foundation for body-mind dynamics.

Our cells not only record all of these stimuli, events, conversations, suspicions, and criticisms that you experience during our life, they also record our reactions to these events, absorbing them as facts regardless of how distorted or out of proportion they may be. Every perceived slight, failure, fright, and inadequacy we've suffered through is embedded in our body's cells, giving rise to anger, frustration, fear, pain, and other feelings whenever something triggers our cellular memories. This is why we may still find our self still mentally replaying unpleasant events from our past, or repeatedly rehashing old grudges. Even if decades have passed and we tell ourselves we no longer care about such things, we will relive the same harmful emotions until we eliminate what causes them— the cellular memories themselves.

Fortunately, over the past 30 or more years a variety of energy-based techniques have been developed that are proving to be very effective for healing unresolved cellular memories and releasing the fears and unhealthy emotions they can cause. Most of these techniques and therapies fall within a relatively new field of energy medicine known as energy psychology. They include therapies you may have heard about such as the emotional freedom technique (EFT), otherwise known as tapping.

A key recommendation is having individuals engage with these therapies with a professional trained in their use. I STRONGLY recommend NOT doing these modalities on your own initially, as results are often better achieved with the active participation and direction of a therapist. For the most part, they work to release stored cellular memories from the body working with acupuncture meridians, the body's energy pathways, in nontraditional ways. They can potentially be quite helpful for resolving stored cellular memories that are causing you stress and negatively impacting your mental and emotional health.

Of these energy psychology techniques, I have found EFT, which was developed by Gary Craig, to be one of the easiest to use, and one of the most effective to release the emotional baggage that holds us back from allowing the energetic shifts that the RCP is designed to allow. It is an ideal technique, especially with a practitioner, for managing stress and healing and releasing our Fe-ars. As those fears, and the not-so-subtle connections to iron, are released, it allows the mineral balancing process in our body to unfold, enhancing all of the other aspects of the Root Cause Protocol. If you are interested in learning more about EFT, you can do so easily online via various EFT websites and instructional YouTube videos.

3) START Donating Blood On A Regular Basis

For men and post-menopausal women, donating blood every three months is the most efficient way to relieve the burden of excess, unbound iron and to jump start our body's "iron REcycling System" (also known as the RES or Reticulo-Endothelial System). Women who are still cycling can obtain these same benefits by donating blood twice a year in addition to their monthly menstrual cycle.

When donating blood, you are donating whole blood, not platelets, plasma, or "power red" donations. In most situations, we can start donating immediately, even before beginning Phase 1 of the RCP. Or you may choose to wait to do so after implementing most or all of Phases 1 - 3 first. Please consider your situation before choosing when to donate.

Each time you donate blood, you eliminate between 225 to 250 mg of iron. In addition to helping to reduce and prevent the buildup of excess, unbound iron in your body, regularly donating blood offers a variety of other important benefits. This includes improving liver function and preventing liver damage caused by excess stored iron. This, in turn, enhances the liver's ability to carry out its more than 500 key enzyme functions, such as blood purification and detoxification, the synthesis of plasma proteins and blood clotting agents, and the metabolism of proteins, fats, and carbohydrates and the nutrients they contain.

Regular blood donation also stimulates the body's ability to produce healthy new blood cells. This is a natural consequence of the body working to replenish blood loss from the donation process. This is a powerful "tonic" to revitalize your metabolism and immune system. The body's ability to heal wounds is also enhanced by regular blood donation because the body's response to replenishing blood loss is similar to its wound healing response. In a sense, by donating blood you are training your body to more efficiently heal wounds, should they occur. Regular blood donation has also been shown to reduce cholesterol and prevent cholesterol from becoming oxidized ("rusting") due to excess iron, thereby reducing the risk of heart disease, especially heart attack and stroke. Donating blood for the same reason can also reduce cancer risk and the risk for most other chronic conditions.

In addition, donating blood can also help our blood flow better, because of how the process reduces blood viscosity (thickness). Thicker blood viscosity places more pressure on the heart because it requires more effort for thick blood to pass through the arteries compared to the effort required for healthy, less thick blood circulation. The flow of thick blood also carries the risk of damaging blood vessels and causing blockages in the arteries, both of which can cause heart attacks. Researchers have found that reducing blood viscosity through regular blood donation can reduce the risk of heart attack by 88 percent. (Salonen JT et al, 1998, Donation of Blood Is Associated with Reduced Risk of Myocardial Infarction. *Am J Epidemiol*, 148(5):44551.)

Finally, and most significantly, every time that you donate blood you are potentially saving lives. According to the National Institutes of Health (NIH), approximately five million Americans require a blood transfusion each year, 20 percent of whom are children. The blood we give during each donation has the potential to help three to four people each time.

It is estimated that only four percent of the entire population of Americans eligible to donate blood do so. I urge you to join their number. For the sake of your health, as well as the health of others. Remember, each pint donated saves four lives: three who benefit from the blood and blood parts, as well as the donor.

To find a blood donation center near you, please contact your local Red Cross (www.redcross.org/give-blood.html), or contact a Blood Center in your local community.

Note: For those who cannot donate blood (due to a medical condition such as history of cancer), ask your doctor to prescribe a "therapeutic phlebotomy" or search for a "mobile phlebotomist" that serves your community or region. They do exist and are increasingly available for this service. They charge a nominal fee, but it is well worth the benefit derived from this donation.

For those who cannot or will not donate or have iron levels that warrant added attention outside of donation, there are a variety of supplemental and food products that can be utilized. Please understand nothing replaces donation but these do offer assistance when donation is not available. Options include: daily apple cider vinegar, turmeric, quercetin, stabilized rice bran, DE, apolactoferrin or a combination product called iDetox which combines apolactoferrin, colostrum, quercetin, bromelain, and a small amount of potassium to facilitate assimilation (for more information or to order, please proceed to http://theirontruth.com)

Additional Considerations: START Getting Exposed To The Right Kinds Of Light

In a very real sense, we are "light beings" and our health and overall wellbeing is derived from the sun. Daily sunlight exposure outdoors provides a multitude of benefits that most doctors ignore and which many people deprive themselves of by routinely spending most of their lives indoors.

What is important to remember is that sunlight ACTIVATES two KEY events:

1) The synthesis (photosynthesis) of vitamin D, and;
2) The breakdown (photocatabolism) of real vitamin A, aka retinol, into a network of retinoids of retinoic acids, and a wide spectrum of nuclear receptors (RARs, RORs, RXRs & RZRs) that support the functions of our nucleic transactions.

It's an irrefutable fact that we human beings are not meant to live our lives cooped up inside our homes and offices, yet that is precisely what so many people are doing each and every day. By contrast, one of the most common traits among people who live long and healthy lives is that they regularly spend time outside in nature, usually on a daily basis. I am convinced that is one of the keys to their notable longevity. Try to get outside in nature for at least 20 to 30 minutes each day. By doing so, we can significantly improve and sustain our health simply by exposing ourselves to sunlight and making direct contact with the earth.

Without the sun, life on Earth would not be possible. Despite this obvious fact, in recent decades we have been taught to fear the sun because scientists and health experts claim sunlight exposure can cause skin cancer. Certainly, we should do all we can to avoid skin cancer, yet failing to obtain the many health benefits regular direct sunlight exposure provides is not the way to go about it.

As with most things in life, moderation is the key. You want to be sure that you do get out in the sun each day, but you don't want to overdo it by developing sunburn. Becoming sunburned on a frequent basis is the real culprit that links sunlight to skin cancer, because sunburn, especially when it is severe, can cause skin cells to mutate, and that's what cancer is—a mutation of otherwise healthy cells.

However, you don't want to use synthetic sunscreens to avoid sunburn. There are two reasons for this. First, the chemicals in such sunscreens can themselves be harmful because they can be absorbed into the skin, where they then enter the bloodstream. Second, synthetic sunscreens, by design, block 95 percent of ultraviolet B (UVB) rays from the sun. UVB rays are what our body needs.

Many scientists now state that retinol was the first hormone on Earth, predating hormone-D by hundreds of millions of years. It turns out that vitamin A is a "light sensor" and, as noted, was a key source of energy (photons), source of information for our vision, and a key indicator of time to regulate the timing of our metabolism. Despite the oft-noted declaration that vitamin D is the "sunshine vitamin," it is really a "light filter" or a "light screen," as I often refer to it, the *"hormone of darkness"* in our cells. Bottom line: vitamin D is essentially the metabolic equivalent of sunglasses! It is NOT the "sunshine vitamin!"

How Regular Sunlight Exposure Benefits our Brain: Regularly getting outdoors and exposing ourselves to natural sunlight provides other health benefits besides ensuring that our body is actively breaking down retinol into retinoids, and producing its own supply of natural vitamin D. Again, this is because of the sun's UV rays. These rays not only enter our body through your skin, but also through our eyes, via both the pupil and the retina. For this reason, it's not wise to wear sunglasses when we go outside.

As discussed in Chapter 9, when the sun's UV rays are absorbed into our eyes, they stimulate the production of dopamine, melatonin, and serotonin, all of which are essential for healthy brain function. Perhaps this is one of the reasons why brain illnesses such as Alzheimer's and dementia are so rare in the long-lived people in what are known as the Blue Zone countries compared to the US and other Western countries.

Here are some guidelines you can follow to ensure that you get all the sunshine you need.

First, make it a point to try and get outdoors every day. The best window of time to expose yourself to the sun is between 10 am to 3 pm. That's because UVA radiation from the sun, which can be harmful and cause skin wrinkling and skin damage, is more pronounced before and after this timeframe.

Depending on your skin color, you may only require 15-20 minutes of sunlight exposure per day, or you may need to stay in the sun for longer periods. If you fall into the latter category you can break up your sunlight exposure times, such as spending 15-20 minutes in the sun during the late morning, and another 15-20 minutes during the afternoon before 3 pm.

Second, understand that for sunlight exposure to be effective, we need to be outside, not facing the sun through a window. Glass (both home and auto) filters out most of the UVB rays that provide benefit to our body. If you wear glasses, please take them off when you obtain sunshine exposure. If you wear contacts, you must also take them out during this time. Wherever possible, please avoid wearing sunglasses.

I realize that getting out in the sun between 10 am and 3 pm is not practical for many folks because of their jobs or other responsibilities. Even so, I encourage you to try to find a way to do so at least a few times a week.

You can also combine joyful movement exercise activities (see below) while being out in the sun. Your ability to get sunlight varies greatly by location, time of year, weather, etc. Just do the best you can to get more sunlight.

Limit Blue Light Radiation Exposure

With increasing frequency, we are inundated with exposure to blue light emissions from our computers, laptops, tablets, cell phones, new model TVs, and LED light bulbs and other LED devices. Once considered safe because sunlight contains blue light wavelengths, researchers now know that excess exposure to blue light, especially during the night, can cause significant health problems. Blue light exposure results in ionizing radiation, which produces hydrogen peroxide.

Hydrogen peroxide, H202, is a significant source of oxidative stress for our eyes and retinas. But our eyes love retinol! Retinol repairs oxidative stress caused by blue light, which is one more reason why it is so important that you supply your body with enough retinol, or real vitamin A, by supplementing with cod liver oil (CLO) each day as recommended in the Root Cause Protocol.

Studies have also confirmed that exposure to blue light at night disrupts circadian rhythm, the body's natural biological clock, and also suppresses the body's production of melatonin. This, in turn, can cause a lack of restorative sleep, as well as insomnia and other sleep conditions. Melatonin is an ancient molecule that is another master antioxidant protein that is actually produced by healthy mitochondria – all over our body. It is not produced just in the pineal gland (Reiter et al, 2014).

Additional studies have also found that blue light exposure can cause or worsen many other diseases, including cancer, depression, diabetes, and heart disease. It is also a factor in obesity, and has been shown to be a major cause of macular degeneration, the leading cause of blindness, that is definitively caused by a dysregulation of copper and iron metabolism that leads to an accumulation of iron and iron-induced oxidative stress.

While exposure to any kind of artificial light at night can suppress melatonin production, the suppression caused by blue light exposure is most pronounced, a fact confirmed by scientific studies. For example, researchers at Harvard University found that 6.5 hours of blue light exposure compared to exposure to light on the green wavelength, aka "sunshine," suppressed melatonin production twice as long and also disrupted circadian rhythms by as much as three hours, compared to a disruption of 1.5 hours caused by light in the green spectrum. Researchers at University of Toledo's (OH) Department of Chemistry and Biochemistry found blue light exposure can also change essential molecules in the retinas of the eyes into cell killers, resulting in age-related macular degeneration.

"We are being exposed to blue light continuously, and the eye's cornea and lens cannot block or reflect it," states Dr. Ajith Karunaratne, assistant professor in the university's Department of Chemistry and Biochemistry. "It's no secret that blue light harms our vision by damaging the eye's retina. Our experiments explain how this happens."

Macular degeneration occurs when photoreceptor cells in the retina die. In order to sense light and trigger the cascade of brain signals associated with vision, these cells require a compound called retinaldehyde. "You need a continuous supply of retinal molecules if you want to see," Dr. Karunarathne explains. "Photoreceptors are useless without retinal."

Dr. Karunarathne and his research colleagues discovered that blue light exposure causes retinal to trigger reactions that generate poisonous chemical molecules in photoreceptor cells. "It's toxic. If you shine blue light on retinal, the retinal kills photoreceptor cells as the signaling molecule on the membrane dissolves," adds Kasun Ratnayake, a PhD student researcher within Dr. Karunaratne's cellular photo chemistry group. "Photoreceptor cells do not regenerate in the eye. When they're dead, they're dead for good." Dr. Karunarathne adds that no such damage is caused by exposure to other light wavelengths. "The retinal-generated toxicity by blue light is universal," he says. "It can kill any cell type."

Given these and other health risk factors caused by blue light, you can see why reducing your exposure to it, particularly at night, is important.

To minimize the harmful effects of blue light you need to take the following precautions:

1. Avoid using electronic devices and looking at your cell phone, computer, laptop, or tablet screens *at least two hours before bedtime.*

2. If you must use electronic devices after sunset, please wear blue light-blocking glasses and install apps on your devices that filter out blue and green wavelength light during nighttime, such as f.lux (www.justgetflux.com), CareUEyes (https://care-eyes.com), or Iris (https://iristech.co). Most of these programs are free to download and work by filtering out blue light emitted from computer and tablet screens.

3. If you work at night, you should also wear blue light-blocking glasses during your shift.

4. Use red lights for night lights. Red light does not disrupt circadian rhythm and suppress melatonin the way that blue light and, to a lesser extent, green light wavelengths do.

5. As much as possible, expose yourself to outdoor sunlight during the day. Doing so can significantly counteract the effects of blue light exposure.

START Doing "Joyful Movement" Exercises

Our body is designed for daily physical activity. However, as a global community, we have become increasingly sedentary, which is one of the primary reasons we now face such a daunting health crisis worldwide. Numerous studies show that sedentary people, on average, don't live as long or enjoy good health to the same degree as those who exercise regularly.

Among the many benefits that research shows regular exercise and physical activity can provide are increased longevity, improved sleep, prevention of serious illness (including heart disease, cancer, and Alzheimer's), stress relief and relief from physical tension, prevention of and relief from anxiety and depression, increased muscular strength and flexibility, improved self-esteem and greater confidence, and increased experiences of positive attitudes and emotions. Regular exercise also aids digestion, increases circulation, and stimulates the lymphatic system (your body's filtration and purification system). Given all of the above benefits, we can see why we need to make regular exercise a priority in your life.

However, many people, when they think of exercise equate it to hard work or drudgery. It needn't be. In fact, the best types of exercises are those that are the most enjoyable. I like to call these forms of exercise "joyful movement." They include activities such as walking, bicycling, swimming, hiking in nature, gardening, or perhaps gently bouncing 15-20 minutes each day on a rebounder (mini-trampoline), if you have one. To the extent that your body can handle it, any form of joyful movement is encouraged on a daily basis.

The Importance of Eating Like Our Ancestors

"Let food be thy medicine and medicine be thy food."
– attributed to Hippocrates, father of Western medicine (460–375 BC)

"No disease that can be treated by diet should be treated by any other means."
– Rabbi Moses Ben Maimon Maimonides (1135–1204 AD)

I agree with the clear focus of both quotations that open this chapter, with one important caveat: Because of how devitalized our crop soil and food supply have become over the last century, as I explained in Chapters 2 and 3, it simply is no longer possible for most people to improve their health by diet alone. That is why I created the Root Cause Protocol, which is the best way I know of for ensuring that we obtain all of the vital minerals, vitamin complexes and other nutrients we require for optimal health and abundant energy, while also keeping iron and oxidative stress in proper check.

At the same time, there is no question that a healthy diet is a crucial cornerstone that must be adhered to as an essential step to building a foundation of lasting vitality and vigor.

But what does such a diet consist of?

In seeking to answer this question I am deeply grateful for and have been greatly influenced by the extensive research conducted by the late Weston A. Price, DDS (1870-1948), and his wife, Florence, who traveled over 100,000 miles in the 1930s to study and document the diets and health of primitive peoples throughout the globe. I consider Dr. Price to be one of the unheralded giants in the history of diet and nutrition, and he is referred to as "the Isaac Newton" of the field. Just as Newton, among his many noteworthy accomplishments, formulated the principle of gravity as a universal force, Price, among his own numerous accomplishments (including discovering, extensively researching, and writing about many of the principles that led to the development of what today is known as holistic dentistry), formulated the basic principles and nutritional components of a healthy diet for humans. Within the RCP, we refer to that as an "Ancestral Diet".

Dr. Price was a highly revered dentist and was determined to discover why so many of his dental patients suffered from dental decay and overall physical degeneration. What specifically fueled his and his wife's passion to engage in a decade of international travel and research to find "perfect teeth" was the tragic and unexpected death of their ten-year-old son, Donald, following a root canal performed by his father. Dr. Price suspected that nutritional deficiencies were the common cause of these dental occurrences. To verify his theory, he and Florence traveled the world for a decade in search of indigenous populations in which healthy teeth and dental arches were most common. He found them in so-called "primitive" cultures and documented 14 such communities, including Native Americans, Eskimos, various African tribes, indigenous peoples in South America, the Aborigines of Australia and the Maori of New Zealand, sea islanders in Polynesia, and isolated communities in rural Switzerland and the Outer Hebrides in Scotland.

All of these groups of people were typically in excellent health, free from most of the diseases of the so-called "civilized world," and they all had healthy, straight teeth, free of cavities and gum disease. Price speculated that their traditional diets were the reason why, and devoted himself to analyzing the foods they ate. What he discovered was that, regardless of where they lived, the foods they consumed, in addition to being fresh and unpreserved, on average had at least four times the mineral content of the foods most Americans were consuming at that time, and at least ten times the amount of vital, fat-soluble vitamins (especially retinol, or real vitamin A) due to their regular consumption of foods such as butter, fish eggs, shellfish and organ meats. (Bear in mind, today the mineral and fat-soluble vitamin content ratios would be even higher in comparison with the standard American diet some 90 years later, due to how devitalized our soil and food have become in the years since Price completed and documented his research.)

The common thread linking the diets of all of the groups Price studied was that they all regularly ate some sort of animal food, whether meats, poultry, fish, and/or shellfish, or insects such as ants (in the case of the Masai tribes of Kenya and Tanzania). In addition, organ meats were commonly part of their diets. Eggs and raw, unpasteurized milk, butter, and other milk products, were also commonly consumed foods.

Meals consisted both of cooked foods and foods eaten raw, and in addition to their rich supply of minerals, vitamins, and healthy fats, the foods also provided these people with an abundant supply of enzymes and beneficial bacteria (probiotics). The fat content of the diet was also quite high at 65 percent, and ranged between 30 to 80 percent of total caloric intake. Healthy saturated and monounsaturated fats predominated in their diets, with less than five percent of the groups' entire fat intake coming from polyunsaturated fats (PUFAs). As a result, the diets also contained a healthy balance of omega-3 and omega-6 fatty acids in an approximate 1:1 ratio. Bones were also part of their diets, being used to create healthy, mineral-rich bone broths that are a rich source of gelatin, which is known to maintain and improve the health of bones and joints in humans, as well as the health of skin and hair. Gelatin also helps to support memory and overall brain function because it contains high amounts of glycine, an amino acid the brain requires in order to stay healthy.

Upon returning to the US, Dr. Price published his findings in his landmark book, *Nutrition and Physical Degeneration*, which is dedicated to his wife, Florence. This text remains in print today despite being widely ignored, unread, and misunderstood by conventional health practitioners. Were this book to be required reading in doctor schools, I am confident that our nation's disease (not health!) crisis could be significantly reversed within a single generation. Since that is unlikely to happen, I recommend you obtain a copy of the book for yourself and your loved ones. I also highly recommend the cookbook *Nourishing Traditions* by Sally Fallon Morell, founding president of the Weston A. Price Foundation and Mary Enig. WAPF is one of the nonprofit organizations that carries on Dr. Price's teachings and work. Her cookbook contains a wonderful assortment of healthy recipes you can use to plan meals that support all of the STARTS of the Root Cause Protocol.

Characteristics of the Ancestral Diet

Though Dr. Price referred to the diets of the people he studied as "traditional," I prefer to call them "ancestral," because this way of eating goes back, mostly unchanged, for thousands of years and was indeed the vitalizing diet of our ancestors.

What follows is a summary of the principles of and guidelines for following the Ancestral Diet. As with the RCP in general, there are both **STOPS** and **STARTS** that you need to follow in order to obtain the full benefits of an ancestral diet. Let's begin with the STOPS. The diets of the peoples that Weston Price studied contained no refined foods. They also were free of ingredients such as refined sugar, high fructose corn syrup, white flour, and pasteurized, homogenized milk. Skim or low-fat milk would also have been unthinkable to these cultures. And, as mentioned, their diets contained very little vegetable oils. You should stop using all such foods and ingredients as well.

In addition, ***all of the following should also be eliminated*** from your diet:

- All "white" carbohydrate foods, including white breads, white pastas, and white rice. (In general, all grains should be avoided or at least greatly minimized in your diet, because of the iron filings they likely contain.)
- All polyunsaturated vegetable (soy, corn, safflower, canola, cottonseed, etc.), hydrogenated, and partially hydrogenated fats and oils. Most restaurants use such oils, instead of healthy oils, which is why I recommend you eat healthy, home-cooked meals as much as possible, and keep dining out to a minimum unless there are restaurants in your area that you know prepare and serve ancestral diet-like meals.
- All foods cooked or fried in polyunsaturated oils.
- All eggs and poultry obtained from factory-farmed, grain-fed chickens.
- All non-free-range meats.
- All farm-raised fish.

- All commercial cereals (including granola).
- All canned foods (except home-canned foods).
- Margarine and all other butter substitutes.
- All GMO (genetically modified) foods, and foods that have been waxed and/or irradiated.
- All food additives, such as MSG, hydrolyzed vegetable protein, aspartame and other artificial sweeteners except stevia or monk fruit (in limited quantities). These ingredients are found in canned soups, sauces, nonorganic broth mixes, and most commercial condiments.
- Also avoid drinking fluoridated tap water, and don't cook with aluminum cookware or microwave ovens. Avoid or minimize buying foods and beverages in the center aisles of grocery stores, as such products are wholly lacking in necessary nutrients.

Finally, despite claims that they are healthy diets, I do not recommend vegetarianism or veganism, as both of these diets lack vital amino acids, and healthy fat soluble vitamins because these nutrients are not found in sufficient quantities in plant foods.

Now let's look at the dietary **STARTS**. As much as you possibly can, please start to do the following:

- Eat whole, unprocessed foods. This should go without saying, but unfortunately far too many folks neglect to do so, to their detriment. Whenever possible, also choose organic foods, ideally from local food sources such as nearby farms and farmers markets.
- Make beef, bison, lamb, poultry, and eggs from grass-fed, free-range animals a staple part of your daily food intake. Also add organ meats, especially liver, at least once per week. Wild-caught fish and shellfish should also be a part of your

weekly food intake because of the wide variety of nutrients they provide. (Farm-raised fish, as mentioned above, should be avoided because of the harmful additives, dyes, and antibiotics such fish are typically laced with. Plus, the foods they are fed are unhealthy, including GMO corn and, often, dog food!)

- If you are not lactose intolerant, milk and other dairy products can also be part of your diet, but be sure to choose these products from pasture-fed cows and goats. Raw milk, whole yogurt, kefir, and cultured butter and cream are all such foods to consider. If you live near Amish communities, you can often obtain foods from Amish farmers. Amish butter is something I especially recommend, enjoy, and use often. When properly made, this butter can contain as much as 90 percent butter fat, compared to conventional brands that are closer to 10 percent. Butter fat is why we eat this delicious dairy product! It is a critical source of fuel for our "fat seeking" and "fat burning" mitochondria.

- Eggs from grass-fed chickens are also highly recommended, including the almost "orange" egg yolks. For decades eggs were considered unhealthy because of their cholesterol content. As is so often the case with medical and governmental dietary recommendations, the "science" behind this warning was incredibly flawed. Eggs from healthy fed and raised chickens are one of the best food sources on the planet because of their nutrient content. Be sure to eat the yolks, which is where much of the nutrients are concentrated. Again, these yolks should be orange, NOT yellow, which means that they have healthy levels of beta-carotenes from the grass in their diet.

- You need to also eat a plentiful supply of fresh, and ideally organic, fruits and vegetables each day. Vegetables are especially important, and can be eaten raw, steamed, or roasted, and also be used in salads and soups. Butter is a critical topping for steamed and roasted vegetables. As Sally Fallon Morell notes in her cookbook and presentations, the real vitamin A (retinol) is the "train" for delivering the nutrients in these vegetables to your body.

- Fermented vegetables, such as sauerkraut, kombucha, and kimchi, are also excellent food sources, and stimulate the production of a far greater amount and variety of healthy bacteria in the gastrointestinal tract than pre- and probiotic supplements are capable of providing. Try to eat fermented foods every day, if possible.

- Seeds and nuts make for excellent energizing snacks during the day. To obtain the most nutritional benefit from them, soak or sprout them first to neutralize the naturally occurring enzyme inhibitors, tannins, and phytic acid they contain in their raw state.

- Overall, low to moderate carbohydrate intake provides the best health outcomes for most people. We all can benefit from carbohydrates to some degree, however. I recommend complex carbohydrates such as legumes (beans), potatoes, sweet potatoes and yams, rather than grains, pastas, and breads.

- I also recommend using only the types of oils used among the cultures Dr. and Mrs. Price explored. Organic, cold-pressed extra virgin olive oil and flaxseed oil are both excellent choices as food toppings and dressings, while organic coconut oil, palm oil and palm kernel oil, as well as butter and lard, are all healthy choices for cooking and sautéing.

- You can also use organic coconut oil to create a healthy alternative to mayonnaise, which is typically made from canola oil (and in some cases corn or soybean oils which are often genetically modified) and other unhealthy ingredients.

- To add flavoring to your meals, please use sea salt or Celtic salt, as well as any organic herbs and spices that you prefer.
- For sweeteners, use organic raw honey, maple syrup, maple sugar, monk fruit, or whole-plant stevia powder, but only sparingly.
- When it comes to beverages, I recommend pure, filtered water as your primary drink (adding in liquid minerals), ideally consumed at least 20 minutes before meals so as not to interfere with your body's digestive process. With meals, sipping organic herbal teas is permitted, as well. Pure, filtered water should also be used when water is required for cooking—making sure to add liquid minerals.
- When cooking, I recommend using only stainless steel, cast iron, glass, or high-quality enamel cookware.

If you enjoy making homemade stocks, do so using bones from free-range meats (beef, lamb, pork), poultry, and wild-caught seafood. You can then use the stocks to make soups, and in stews, gravies, and sauces. Also, a cup of warm, salted bone broth is a nice snack, and is especially good when you feel "under the weather."

Increase Your Energy by Intermittent Fasting

A growing body of research is showing that limiting the window of time in which you eat each day can help keep you healthier and might even extend your life. Known as time restricted eating, or intermittent fasting, this approach means consuming all of the foods you eat each day within an eight to 12-hour period. By doing so, you allow your body 12 to 16 hours to rest and repair itself through a process known as autophagy.

Derived from the Greek words *auto*, ("self") and *phagein* ("to eat"), autophagy is a natural process of cellular cleansing in which the body essentially "eats" parts of itself by breaking down and then eliminating old, worn down proteins, cell membranes, and other parts of cells which can no longer be sustained by the body's energy. This enables the body to replace and/or recycle these cellular components with new, healthier versions, thereby helping the body to maintain itself.

Autophagy can only occur during times of fasting, which time restricted eating mimics to some extent. Time restricted eating is not the same thing as dieting or calorie restriction. You can eat as you normally would as long as you limit the window of time each day in which you do so.

We can further increase the benefits autophagy provides by periodically fasting. A 24-hour water fast done weekly or every other week is safe for most people to undergo. In addition to enabling cell cleansing, fasting has also been shown to stimulate the body's production of growth hormones, which typically decline as we age. You may also wish to explore periodic longer fasts of three to five days, although these should initially be undertaken under the supervision of a doctor or other health practitioners familiar with fasting's known therapeutic benefits.

While the idea of intermittent fasting may seem foreign, even unnatural, to you, this is actually the eating method that many of our ancient ancestors followed as hunter-gatherers. In fact, evidence suggests that these nomadic peoples were able to maintain the health they required in order to stay alive in those times while often eating only one meal a day, usually in the evening, after a day spent foraging and hunting for food. I'm not recommending that we only eat one meal a day, but I do recommend that we consider experimenting with time restricted eating. As always, let your body be your guide and pay attention to how you feel after a few weeks or more. You may find that it enhances the benefits that following an ancestral diet provides.

Final Thoughts

As with everything else related to the Root Cause Protocol, when it comes to adopting an ancestral diet, remember that it is direction, nor perfection, that we seek to aim for. There is no perfection when it comes to diet, any more than there is perfection in any other aspect of our lives. What matters is continuing to move forward in the direction of health. At times, we may wish to indulge in a non-ancestral food, such as a pizza, an ice cream, or a slice of pie. If so, do so with pleasure every once and a while, confident that the overall foundation of health you are creating by following the precepts of the RCP can more than compensate for such occasional lapses or "indulgences."

Overall, the idea of the Ancestral Diet is very simple, yet very powerful because of how following it leads to improved health and more energy. It can be summarized in three words: *Eat real food!* Get in the habit of doing so more and more each day, until it becomes fully integrated into your daily lifestyle.

Part of that lifestyle, as my friend and colleague, Ben Edwards, MD points out, involves slowing down and taking time to fully enjoy our healthy meals instead of rushing through them. Restricting your intake of food obtained through your car window is a must! It also involves, if possible, spending time getting to know the local farmers in your area and learning where your food really comes from, shopping at the right places to obtain all of the ingredients needed, and then taking the time to prepare meals, recognizing that doing so is a way to honor ourselves and take care of the body our Creator blessed us with. By connecting all of these dots, as it were, we will truly come to understand that our food really is our medicine.

But, of course, the health improvements the ancestral diet provides will not occur overnight. As I share with my clients, Aesop's fable is true: *The tortoise always wins.* That can be difficult for some people to accept, because we all have the "impatience gene," especially people who have been chronically ill or who have suffered from prolonged fatigue. It's human nature to want to get well yesterday. However, healing rarely works that way. In traditional Chinese medicine, it is said that every year that one has been sick requires one month of cure. I find there is a lot of truth in that statement.

Doing this work for as long as I have working with clients, I also have found that the longer it takes a person to get back to balance and regain their health and energy, the longer those gains will last. (Please re-read that sentence, again.) We all need to appreciate the very measured, steady pace that healing involves because that is how the body is designed to achieve and maintain its homeostasis. So, commit yourself to the RCP lifestyle, including the ancestral diet. I hate to even use the word "diet," but I really have to because, by default, most people are eating the standard American diet, even if they don't realize it, and it's literally stealing away their health and vitality and accelerating their metabolic demise. That is why returning to the foods and eating practices of our Ancestors is so very important.

Happy, healthy eating or as I so often say online, ***A vôtre santé!***

12

Frequently Asked Questions (FAQs)

"The important thing is not to stop questioning. Curiosity has its own reason for existing."

– Albert Einstein

"Curiosity is, in great and generous minds, the first passion and the last."

– Samuel Johnson

What follows are a representative sampling of the many questions that are routinely asked by those practicing the recommendations of the Root Cause Protocol. This list is by no means exhaustive and the RCP website (see Resources) has a more up-to-date and complete list of the questions posed and answered over the years. **https://therootcauseprotocol.com/all-resources/**

"How long will it take for the Root Cause Protocol to work?"

The truth is, "it depends." The time it takes is based on how your body reacts to each nutrient that is part of the Root Cause Protocol, and also depends on the extent to which you believe in your body's natural ability to rebuild and rebalance itself. There are numerous nutritional and emotional dimensions to this recovery process.

To give you a range, the "course record" is a woman who implemented all of the STOPS and the STARTS within a few weeks and experienced dramatic changes within 60 days. But then there are others who've taken 18 months or longer to implement the STARTS because their body needed that much time to detoxify and acclimate. Your mileage will vary. Listen to your body and please remember that it is a process. And despite your desire to "get well yesterday," this natural process does take time, discipline, devotion and a dash of patience.

"How long do I need to follow these steps?"

The Root Cause Protocol is a lifestyle change — your body will always need minerals like magnesium and whole food vitamin complexes like A, C, E, etc.

The STARTS are designed to be followed indefinitely as they supply the key nutrients missing in today's modern diet, laden with refined and processed foods. How quickly or slowly you decide to implement each of the STARTS is up to you, and how well your body responds to each substance that is introduced and incorporated. The Protocol that is readily available on our website has suggested Phases that many have found to be a useful guide to this process.

> *"I have been told I'm anemic, now what? I tested low in iron and this protocol wants to increase copper to decrease unbound iron, so how does that solve anemia? I have low iron, what do I do? I've been taking supplements for low iron, but now I hear that I shouldn't be doing this, what do I do instead?"*

Questions like those above are very frequently asked by people new to the Root Cause Protocol. It is important to have the full context of whether or not you have true iron deficiency or whether it is more likely masquerading as "anemia of chronic disease" or "anemia of inflammation" – different names for the SAME condition caused by a LACK of bioavailable copper. Iron in the body is designed to be in circulation, to be moving, and to *not* be stored. Generally, the blood tests for iron status used by practitioners are showing iron in the blood, and *not showing iron status actually stored in the tissue.* Often these tests use incomplete markers or are not looking at other important connections to the "low iron in the tissue" aspect.

If you have low iron in the blood, it is very likely that you have high-unbound iron in the tissues, organs, etc. which signals a lack of bioavailable copper.

The Root Cause Protocol aims at reconnecting the unbound iron to its transport protein, transferrin, by increasing ceruloplasmin (bioavailable copper). Transferrin and ceruloplasmin are the "fric and frac" of ensuring optimal circulation of iron. For instance, if you have had your ferritin tested, it is a marker, which doesn't accurately reflect your storage of iron inside the cells. Far and away, hemoglobin is a better marker given that it represents 70% of the body's iron stores, but even when it is low, there is more going on than just you not having enough iron. The MOST important question that is NOT adequately addressed in standard blood tests is: *Is this iron functional, doing what it is designed to do?* Simple "high," vs "low" metrics are NOT comprehensive enough given the known complexities of iron circulation.

If you want further personalized help, consider doing the blood tests discussed in Chapter 6 and a hair tissue mineral analysis and then obtaining help from either myself or one of the RCP consultants. (For a directory of consultants, please see the Resources section in this book.)

"Can I use magnesium citrate to maintain my body's magnesium levels?

No, magnesium citrate is not recommended on the protocol for two principal reasons:

1) The citrate molecule irritates the bowel and prevents sufficient time for magnesium to get absorbed.
2) The citrate molecule causes the ceruloplasmin (ferroxidase) protein to lose its enzyme function. (Osaki S et al, 1964-Jan, Citric Acid as the Principal Serum Inhibitor of Ceruloplasmin. *Jrl Biol Chem*; 239(1): PC364-365.)

Without sufficient levels of the ceruloplasmin ferroxidase enzyme functioning properly, our bodies cannot oxidize the iron and load that iron onto transferrin so that the iron can be transported through the blood to where it is needed and eventually taken back to the bone marrow and recycled to make new heme, hemoglobin and ultimately red blood cells. Therefore, due to low ceruloplasmin ferroxidase enzyme function, the unbound iron will simply not be functional, and will "appear" low in the blood. Again, as we noted previously, every second of every day, we need to make between 2-3 million new red blood cells to replace those that are completing their 120-day life cycle. This iron cycle is profoundly important and is largely directed and regulated by bioavailable copper. The fact that your doctor does not know this, but it is clearly documented in the research should be an added point of curiosity for you.

"What types of magnesium are recommended?"

There are many different types of magnesium which we can benefit from. On the RCP, we encourage a diversity of different forms of magnesium; one type of magnesium is not better than the other, it is individual to what you may tolerate and benefit from. We do recommend you start with mineral drops, as these can be added in slowly. The adrenal cocktail is also very important to take when you are taking magnesium, especially in the initial stages of the Protocol. It helps to support your electrolyte balance when taking supplemental magnesium.

There are four categories of recommended magnesium:

> **Food**: Among the best food sources of magnesium are leafy greens (beet greens, collard greens, mustard greens, etc.), nuts (especially cashews and almonds), pumpkin seeds, and spinach. There are clearly other food sources, as well.
>
> **Water**: Magnesium bicarbonate (Mag Water), one of the co-factors, improves absorption. (The recipe for this form of magnesium is available in the Resources section.)
>
> **Transdermal**: Magnesium Chloride (aka, Mg Oil), can be used transdermally on skin or in baths, and is found in mineral drops. Magnesium sulfate (aka Epsom Salts) is a wonderful form of magnesium for detoxifying and relieving muscle aches and strains.

Chelated Magnesium Supplements

Magnesium Glycinate – often calming, so a good one for nighttime use.

Magnesium Malate – can be a stimulating magnesium, so good for start of the day.

Magnesium Taurate and Orotate – good forms of magnesium for cardiovascular health.

Magnesium Threonate– a recognized form to cross the blood brain barrier for brain injuries, PTSD, depression, neurological conditions, and anxiety (though many other types of magnesium can and do cross the blood brain barrier, it is individual to what you may tolerate and utilize).

Keep in mind that, although magnesium is critically important, it is the copper-iron conflict in the body that affects the production of oxidative stress that then causes relentless loss of magnesium in our cells and tissues. Please understand the following:

Restoring magnesium loss SOLVES symptoms.

Restoring bioavailable copper CORRECTS the problem CAUSING magnesium loss.

That is a notable difference, and is why the focus of the Root Cause Protocol is on resolving the copper-iron dynamic so that our body has all of the bioavailable copper it needs to both create energy and clear exhaust.

"What can I do for anxiety?"

Please know that, on a physical, biochemical level, all forms of anxiety are a result of iron-induced oxidative stress. The Root Cause Protocol corrects this underlying metabolic problem. In addition, you can address the non-physical aspects of anxiety using the Emotional Freedom Techniques (EFT) discussed in Chapter 10.

"What can I do for migraines?"

Many people have found that implementing the RCP has helped with migraines, especially because of the magnesium supplementation and adrenal cocktails that are a key part of the protocol. If you suffer from migraine or headache, you should also make sure that you get plenty of potassium-rich food sources in your diet.

Copper dysregulation that leads to excess oxidative stress are behind many migraines. The RCP aims at increasing bioavailable copper and is designed to help reduce this oxidative stress. Magnesium's role is to respond to the oxidative stress, so often just magnesium alone can help, but doing the full protocol helps to restore the mineral and metabolic balance so migraines are significantly reduced. Metabolic and emotional stressors are also implicated because they trigger magnesium loss, which then can trigger migraines.

"I'm pregnant and have been told that I have low iron. How can the Root Cause Protocol help me?"

The Root Cause Protocol (RCP) is ideal during pregnancy, as well as during breastfeeding. The only exclusions from the RCP are diatomaceous earth (DE) and stabilized rice bran, since we do not know the effects they might have on the baby due to their detoxification effects. Minerals are vitally important for pregnant and breastfeeding mothers. We openly challenge the assertion that "anemia of iron deficiency" exists, and we focus on the lack of functional iron, which is a very different perspective. The RCP is designed to make our copper bioavailable which will enable the iron to get functional.

An important caution is to **not** use a ferritin-only blood test to determine iron status as it is not fully representative of iron's true status. It takes bioavailable copper, as expressed via ferroxidase enzyme function, which lowers as the pregnancy progresses. We need bioavailable copper to load iron into ferritin. Therefore, low ferroxidase means low ferritin. We need more bioavailable copper, not more iron.

Normal hemoglobin (Hgb) for women is 12.5-13.5. When a woman is pregnant, this level stays the same for the first half of the pregnancy. During the second half of the pregnancy, Hgb should drop to between 8.5-9.5 (Steer PJ et al, 1995). This drop in hemoglobin status is called hemodilution, it is also known as "anemia of pregnancy." *It is NOT a sign of LOW iron in the blood, but a sign of HIGH innate intelligence in the mother's body.*

According to Philip J. Steer, MD, who examined 150,000 live births, "Maximum mean birth weight in women was achieved with a lowest hemoglobin concentration in pregnancy of 85-95 g/l [8.5-9.5 g/dL]; the lowest incidence of low birth weight and preterm labor occurred with a lowest hemoglobin of 95-105 g/l [9.5-10.5 g/dL]." (Steer P. et al, 1995-Feb25, Relation between maternal hemoglobin concentration and birth weight in different ethnic groups. BMJ; 310: 489-491) Dr. Steer's research confirms that the babies with the healthiest weight are born to mothers with hemoglobin lower than what is found in non-pregnant healthy women.

Copper levels in pregnant women can be difficult to assess, as ceruloplasmin, a key protein for copper as we've learned, is very high because mothers are supposed to engage in a notable download of copper into the fetus's liver during the last trimester. This is true of all mammals. It is also worth knowing that there are three forms of ferroxidase enzyme that express in the mother's womb throughout the pregnancy: ceruloplasmin, hephaestin and zyklopen, this last form of bioavailable copper, is mostly found in the placenta throughout the pregnancy. All are engaged in the regulation, circulation and utilization of iron in the pregnant mom and the developing fetus. None are measured in conventional obstetrics and midwifery. You might ask your birthing practitioner why that is the case. In a word, I find it alarming.

Cod liver oil is a wonderful source of retinol, which is essential to enable a key copper-pumping enzymes to work so that the master anti-oxidant protein, ceruloplasmin, is properly loaded with copper and is fully functional to perform its many antioxidant functions. This protein and its ferroxidase enzyme expression, is key to the proper and natural regulation of iron and oxygen in the human body, as well as dozens of other anti-oxidant functions. Vitamin A toxicity is usually due to synthetic supplemental vitamin A, not from food sources such as unfortified cod liver oil, grass fed beef liver, grass fed butter, eggs, and heavy cream. It is difficult to stress just how important animal-based retinol (vitamin A) is. Retinol is designed by MTHR Nature to be downloaded via mother's breast milk during the first 18-24 months of the newborn baby's life.

The Root Cause Protocol helps to ensure that all of the above conditions are met.

"I'm pregnant and my hemoglobin is low. How do I raise my hemoglobin?"

As we learned from Dr. Steer, the need for increased hemoglobin is not the correct focus during the course of the pregnancy. The factors that are far more important are:

- Retinol has proven properties to increase Hgb (likely by dual effect on lowering H2O2 and making copper more bioavailable).
- Bioavailable copper is involved in 4 of the 8 enzymes to make heme, especially the first (rate-limiting) and last, where copper is the "crane-operator" in the ferrochelatase enzyme to insert iron into heme. (*Iron does not "insert" itself!*)
- Bioavailable copper is key to making anti-oxidant enzymes, especially, ferroxidase, SOD, catalase and GPx that must be optimal to make Hgb. More iron only increases the "accidents with oxygen," aka "oxidants" that must then be neutralized.
- Another key requirement to make new blood (Heme >> Hgb >> RBCs) is energy. Erythroid cells, the precursor cells to red blood cells, with low bioavailable copper cannot make optimal energy and therefore are not able to differentiate into the more mature form of the red blood cell.

Oh, how I wish your doctor had been trained in what I'm sharing with you here. The reason why RCP consultants do not use or recommend "heme iron tablets" or FeSO4 tablets is because we understand the truth of blood metabolism— not the scripted understanding that is based solely on a grade-school dipstick measurements of "high" vs "low" levels of iron.

Copper<>iron metabolism is among the MOST sophisticated and MOST intricate aspects of human physiology. The profound and subtle aspects of their homeostasis have been REDUCED to child-like measurement of "high" and "low" factors. Nothing could be farther from the truth. What the research teaches us and what we are sharing with you here is that iron is either *functional* or it is *stuck*!

"What if I'm pregnant or nursing?"

All of the RCP steps are recommended during pregnancy EXCEPT for diatomaceous earth, stabilized rice bran, and donating blood. Those can be introduced AFTER you've stopped nursing.

Also, we always encourage that you share this Root Cause Protocol with your doctor or midwife so that you are both on the same page, and so that your birthing practitioner can be educated on the mineral dynamics of the RCP if they are not aware of this protocol already.

"What about other supplements like Co-Q10, probiotics, etc? Should I stop everything that isn't on the Root Cause Protocol?"

If a particular item is not listed in the STOPS or the STARTS that means I've not read enough peer-reviewed research to establish an official position either way. But my passion in life is reading scientific literature. (*Yes, I'm quite the nerd these days!*) So, as we uncover new steps, and as we learn what is working best in the RCP community, the protocol will be updated, and you'll receive an email notifying you of changes. In the meantime, please consider joining the premium RCP Community and posing your non-RCP product specific questions there. The RCP Community is filled with many who have been implementing RCP in their own lives, and they likely have experience with the product you wish to know about.

"What if I'm vegetarian or vegan?"

Unfortunately, there is no way to fully implement the RCP and remain vegetarian or vegan because there are no plant-based sources of retinol (wholefood vitamin A). And retinol from animal sources (primarily, cod liver oil and beef liver) are deemed central for increasing bioavailable copper (and thus, ensuring functional iron), which is the entire focus of the RCP. Vitamin A (as beta-carotene) from plant sources is decidedly different from retinol. Beta-carotene, alone, does not increase bioavailable copper. Please see this article from a third party at the following link for more information on this topic. (https://empoweredsustenance.com/truevitamin-a-foods/)

"What about MTHFR and epigenetics? How do they relate to the Root Cause Protocol?"

It's very vogue and hip to talk about methylation. But truth be known, most health practitioners and know very little about the truth of this metabolic condition and how impacted it is from choline deficiency, copper deficiency and iron-induced oxidative stress.

Lack of bioavailable copper affects the methyltransferase enzymes that our genes and DNA rely upon.

My friend and colleague, Kitty Martone, runs a very popular and informative Facebook group on estrogen dominance. In her formative years as a nutritionist, she spent many years working with Robert Marshall, MD, who specializes in gut health and pH balance. What they learned in his center, through regular 23andMe testing, is that the "methylation issues" that surfaced on initial MTHFR testing changed and improved as the metabolic health of the client improved.

Now that is an absolute bombshell, and confirms what I have long suspected: Genes flip "on" and "off" all the time, depending on the metabolic load and stressors of the individual. And no one ever thinks to "test their 'broken' genes" again. So, as the mineral dysregulation that's at the head of all this chaos subsides, the stress on the genes changes and metabolic function improves. This is what the RCP can help you accomplish.

"Though the Root Cause Protocol makes good sense to me, I find the thought of implementing it for myself overwhelming! Can I talk to someone?"

Yes, you can. If you have any questions about how to best implement certain steps of the RCP for yourself or a loved one, you can get personalized help from an expert RCP Consultant. You will find a list of consultants in the Resources section of this book.

"I LOVE what RCP has done for me, how can I support this cause?"

Please contact RCP Customer Service and share your success story with us so that we may add you to the ever-growing list of Root Cause Protocol Testimonials. You can do so here: https://therootcauseprotocol.com/contact.

Also, please consider joining the Premium RCP Community to get exclusive access to new, ongoing research, to collaborate with others who are following the RCP, and much more! You can sign up at https://therootcauseprotocol.com/join-community.

Most importantly, we would ask that you "pay it forward" and share these concepts with your family, friends, and those open to these enduring concepts that will be willing to take personal control over their health. The steps of the RCP are "simple," but they are not necessarily "easy." A key way to support this cause is to support those seeking to adopt these ancient principles of nutrition and vitality.

Resources

There is general resource information, as well as helpful charts for implementing the RCP on the dedicated book website:

https://cureyourfatiguebook.com/resources

In addition, the following options are available to you if you would like help implementing the Root Cause Protocol, or if you wish to deepen your understanding of the RCP:

https://therootcauseprotocol.com

This is the main website for the RCP, where you will find a lot of free information.

https://therootcauseprotocol.com/rcpc-directory

This is the website directory of RCP consultants around the world who have been trained by Morley Robbins. They are available to help you or your loved ones implement the RCP and to answer any questions you may have.

https://therootcauseprotocol.com/get-help-from-morley

This is the website link to use if you wish to book a one-on-one consultation with Morley Robbins.

https://therootcauseprotocol.com/rcp-101-video-series

This is the website for the RCP 101 Video Series, an online instruction site that goes into further depth about the WHY behind each step of the RCP. It is available for a one-time purchase of $99 and backed by a 30-day money-back guarantee.

https://therootcauseprotocol.com/join-community

The website of the RCP membership community. This premium community is a place for sharing tips about the RCP, and for asking questions about how to get the most out of RCP and to get other supplement and health advice. Here you can also learn about new research uncovered by the creator of the RCP, Morley Robbins, including live Q&A webinars 1-2 times each month. Both Morley and other RCP Consultants (the RCP experts!) are regular contributors to this community. By joining, you'll get to interact and learn from others who are implementing the RCP into their own lives. You'll also get exclusive access to new RCP research, and much more!

https://therootcauseprotocol.com/rcp-institute

If you'd like to become a "Mineral Detective," sign up to attend the RCP Institute, which offers a guided journey to better health, with classes taught by Morley Robbins, the creator of the RCP. Students who complete this training also have the opportunity to become certified as RCP Consultants.

https://www.facebook.com/RootCauseProtocol

A free Facebook group site founded by Morley Robbins, at which he shares his latest research, videos, and which acts as a forum for others to discuss their own experiences with the RCP and have their questions answered.

https://www.facebook.com/groups/MagnesiumAdvocacy

Home of the Magnesium Advocacy Group discussing the Root Cause Protocol, this free group site was founded by Morley Robbins to be a place where anyone interested in learning more about the RCP can ask questions and share tips.

About the Author

"Two roads diverged in a woods and I – I took the one less traveled by, and that has made all the difference."
– Robert Frost

Morley M. Robbins, MBA, CHC, is the creator of the Root Cause Protocol. Also known as "Magnesium Man," he is one of the foremost experts on magnesium's role in the body, and the delicate dance magnesium plays with iron, copper, and calcium. He received his BA in Biology from Denison University in Ohio, and holds an MBA from George Washington University in healthcare administration, with additional concentrations in finance and marketing management. Morley has completed his training for becoming a WellCoaches Wellness Coach, a Ulan Nutritional Counselor, a Functional Diagnostic Nutritionist, and completed two levels of Jerry Tennant, MD's Synergy Institute.

In 2012, Morley founded the Magnesium Advocacy Group, and remains the de facto leader of the Magnesium Advocacy Group on Facebook, with almost 200,000 members (and growing weekly). As a certified health coach with an expertise in Hair Tissue Mineral

Analysis (HTMA), Morley has performed over 6,500 one-on-one consultations with clients from 45 countries around the world.

Morley has a mainstream medical industry background. He had been a hospital executive and consultant for 32 years when in the Fall of 2008, he developed a condition called "frozen shoulder." His family doctor recommended surgery as the only hope for Morley if he wanted to be able to lift his right hand above his waist ever again. Friends who owned a health food store intervened and encouraged Morley to try chiropractic care. His initial response: *"Thanks guys, but I don't do witchcraft."*

Several months later, the pain was unrelenting and continuing to wear on him, and his health food friends insisted. It only took a couple weeks of "light touch chiropractic care" (Network Spinal Analysis) before his shoulder had full range of motion once again.

The experience was so life-changing for Morley, he questioned everything he knew—or thought he knew—about healing. He left the world of hospital administration and dove deep down the rabbit hole of natural healing, never to look back.

In July 2009, Morley read Carolyn Dean's wonderful book *The Magnesium Miracle*. He realized that this was a key piece of the health puzzle that virtually no practitioners seemed to be aware of—even in the natural health world. He was captivated by this mineral, and went on to read even more. Much, much more.

After reading scores of books and thousands of scientific studies and articles (*and counting daily*), Morley has come to realize what the scientific, peer-reviewed literature from around the world makes very clear—even though it is not well known in conventional medical circles: All disease is caused by inflammation, better described as "oxidative stress." And the root cause of this inflammation/oxidative stress is "cellular metabolic dysfunction" which is caused by an imbalance and dysregulation of three key minerals: copper, magnesium, and iron.

This imbalance can be repaired—and we can feel much better—following the steps of the Root Cause Protocol. Spreading the news about these mineral truths is now Morley's full-time mission. He views it as his life's work to push back the tides of nutritional insanity, supplemental iron, and is fully committed to educating as many people as possible about how they can use the RCP to reverse this "root cause" mineral imbalance and end the plague of fatigue that fuels chronic disease throughout the world.

Made in the USA
Middletown, DE
19 August 2022

71408474R00176